Richard Brennan STAT, MATI is a member of Alexander Technique International, runs a busy Alexander Technique practice in Galway Ireland, and numerous adult education classes and other courses throughout the British Isles and Europe. He also gives talks and lectures at various schools, colleges and universities, for the press and radio, and at health and healing exhibitions. He has been a pioneer in helping to make the technique accessible to many thousands of people. He is currently in the process of setting up the first Alexander technique teacher training college in Ireland.

ALSO BY RICHARD BRENNAN

Health Essentials: The Alexander Technique
The Alexander Technique Manual

The Alexander Technique Workbook

YOUR PERSONAL PROGRAMME FOR HEALTH, POISE AND FITNESS

RICHARD BRENNAN

E L E M E N T

Shaftesbury, Dorset ● Boston Massachusetts
Melbourne, Victoria

© Element Books Limited 1992
Text © Richard Brennan 1992

First published in Great Britain in 1992 by
Element Books Limited
Shaftesbury, Dorset SP7 8BP

Published in the USA in 1992 by
Element Books, Inc.
160 North Washington Street,
Boston, MA 02114

Published in Australia in 1992 by
Element Books
and distributed by Penguin Australia Limited
487 Maroondah Highway, Ringwood, Victoria, 3134

Reprinted June 1993
Reprinted January, April, October and December 1994
Reprinted 1995
Reprinted February and July 1996
Reprinted 1997
Reprinted 1998 (twice)

Cover design by Max Fairbrother
Cover illustration by David W. Hamilton/Image Bank
Design by Roger Lightfoot
Illustrations by David Gifford
Typeset by BP Intergraphics Ltd, Bath, Avon
Printed and bound in Great Britain by
J W Arrowsmith Limited, Bristol, Avon

British Library Cataloguing in Publication data available

Library of Congress Cataloguing in Publication Data
Brennan, Richard.
    The Alexander technique workbook/Richard Brennan.
        p.   cm.
    Includes bibliographical references and index.
    ISBN 1-85230-346-8 (pb): $14.95
    1. Alexander technique.   I. Title
RA781.5.B74 1992
615.8'2—dc20   92-28403
                                                    CIP

ISBN 1-85230-346-8

CONTENTS

TO BE WHAT WE ARE
AND TO BECOME WHAT
WE ARE CAPABLE OF
BECOMING IS THE
ONLY END OF LIFE.

Robert Louis Stevenson

This book is dedicated to
all those who have the
courage to take the risks
necessary to discover their
True Self.

INTRODUCTION

The Alexander Technique is a method of releasing the physical and mental tensions that many of us have accumulated throughout our lives. Often we are unaware of these tensions until we become ill and are unable to go on. They can contribute to headaches, backache, heart problems, arthritis and depression, as well as a whole range of ailments too numerous to mention. If these unconscious muscular tensions are allowed to continue, as they often are, they can affect our quality of life by accelerating the ageing process and decreasing our vitality.

The ease and grace with which we move slowly become lost as we take on more burdens and responsibilities. The Alexander Technique can help us to regain that poise and ease during even the most simple tasks. Our body is our most precious possession, yet we tend to give it the least attention – apart from when we are trying to look attractive. Without knowing it, we grossly interfere with our natural flow of movement to such an extent that many of us will at some time in our lives suffer from backache, solely due to poor posture. Yet there is nothing more attractive than someone who is moving in a balanced and co-ordinated way.

Few people are aware that the Alexander Technique exists, and as a result many millions of people every year suffer needlessly. In this book I hope to explain the Alexander Technique as simply as possible, and through simple observation exercises and procedures to show clearly how it can help you to enjoy a happier and more fulfilling life.

ACKNOWLEDGEMENTS

I would like to thank Caroline Green for her constant support and help with the writing of this book. I would also like to thank Susan Mears and Valerie Finlay of Element Books for their efforts during all the stages of the production of this book.

Chapter 1

In the Beginning

Imagination is more important than knowledge.
ALBERT EINSTEIN

When beginning to learn the Alexander Technique for yourself, it is important to follow, step by step, Alexander's own discoveries about himself and the way he developed this method of teaching other people. But first I wish to describe the steps leading up to his discovery.

A LITTLE HISTORY

Frederick Matthias Alexander was born in Australia on 20th January 1869. He began life and spent his childhood in Wynyard, a small town on the north-west coast of Tasmania. The eldest of eight children born to John and Betsy Alexander, Frederick was born prematurely and was not expected to live more than a few weeks. It was only his mother's overwhelming love for her child that ensured his survival. (She was in fact the local nurse and midwife.)

Throughout his childhood, Frederick was plagued with one illness or another, mainly asthma and other respiratory difficulties. Although he started school, he was soon taken away through ill-health and given private tuition in the evenings by the village school teacher. This left him with plenty of free time during the day to spend with his father's horses. Gradually he became expert at training and managing them and in this way acquired the sensitivity of touch which was to prove invaluable later on.

At the age of nine or ten Frederick's health began to

improve, and at seventeen financial pressures within the family forced him to leave the outdoor life he had grown to love, to work in the office of a tin-mining company in the nearby town of Mount Bischoff. In his spare time he developed an interest in amateur dramatics and playing the violin.

By the time he was twenty he had saved up enough money to travel to Melbourne where he stayed with his uncle, and for three months spent all his hard-earned money experiencing the best in theatre, art, and music. By the end of that time he had decided to train as a reciter.

To finance his training, which he did in the evenings and at weekends, Frederick took various jobs: working in an estate agent's office, in a large department store, and even as a tea taster for a firm of tea merchants. He quickly established an excellent reputation as an actor and reciter, and soon formed his own theatre company, specializing in one-man Shakespeare recitals. He was particularly fond of *The Merchant of Venice* and *Hamlet*.

Before long, the respiratory troubles that had plagued Frederick as a young child returned. His voice became hoarse; and on one particular occasion he completely lost his voice during a performance. Soon he was reluctant to accept engagements for fear of losing his voice at a crucial moment in front of an audience. Seeking advice from doctors and voice trainers, he was given medication and was instructed to rest his voice, and to gargle. But these solutions gave only temporary relief.

The career he loved was in jeopardy, and he was willing to try anything to find a cure. Finally one of his doctors prescribed a complete rest of the voice for a full two weeks before his next recital. The doctor assured him that if he followed these instructions to the letter his voice would return to normal.

By this time Frederick was so desperate that he hardly spoke at all during that time, and by the beginning of his recital the hoarseness had completely disappeared. Halfway through the programme, however, his voice was again 'in the most distressing condition', and by the end of the evening the hoarseness was so acute that he could hardly speak. His disappointment was beyond words when he realized he could never look forward to more than temporary relief, and would thus be forced to give up a career to which he was deeply committed, and which promised to be highly successful.

The next day he went back to the same doctor whose only advice was that he should persevere with the treatment. 'But', said Frederick, 'if my voice was perfect at the beginning of my recital, yet had deteriorated so much that by the end I could barely speak, is it not fair to conclude that it was something I was doing that evening in using my voice that was the cause of the trouble?'

The doctor thought for a moment, and then agreed, thus prompting Frederick to enquire: 'Can you tell, then, what it was I did that caused the trouble?' The doctor frankly admitted that he could not. 'Very well, if that is so,' Frederick replied, 'I must try and find out for myself.'

This dialogue between Frederick Alexander and his doctor is at the heart of the technique he was to go on to develop. It was his conviction that if we suffer from headaches, backache, arthritis, insomnia, or other ailments, there must always be a cause at the root of the problem. He was applying the well-known physical law of cause and effect: that every action has an opposite reaction.

Alexander had experienced the reaction as the loss of his voice. Now he needed to discover the action that was causing this phenomenon.

DEVELOPING THE TECHNIQUE

A detailed description of how Alexander developed his Technique can be found in the next chapter. He in fact spent many years examining himself minutely in front of mirrors to detect the exact reason for the hoarseness in his voice.

After finding the solution to his problem, word soon spread about Alexander's success in 'curing' himself, and many actors and reciters began to seek his advice. He began to realize that with the gentle guidance of his hands he could correct other people's many and varied ailments.

Although he resumed his career of acting and reciting, he also began to take on pupils and to teach them his Technique on a professional basis. At this point he was joined by his younger brother, Albert Redden Alexander, and together they worked out various procedures and instructions which were incorporated into the Technique. The two brothers worked together for about six years, teaching in Sydney and Melbourne.

The practice continued to grow as the emphasis began to shift away from voice development and on to the control of reactions throughout the whole body; and several doctors began referring their patients to the Alexander brothers. One of them, Doctor J. W. Stewart McKay, a prominent surgeon in Sydney, persuaded Frederick to go to London in order to bring the Technique before a larger public.

He left Australia for good in the spring of 1904, and with only a reference of introduction from Doctor McKay, he soon set up a practice in Victoria Street, and later moved to 16 Ashley Place, in the centre of London.

Alexander had little difficulty establishing his teaching methods, and became something of a cult figure. He taught many prominent figures, amongst them George Bernard Shaw, Aldous Huxley, Sir Henry Irving (actor), Sir Charles Sherrington (Nobel prizewinner for physiology and medicine), and Professor E. Coghill (anatomist and physiologist).

He continued to practise in London until war broke out in 1914, when he set sail for the United States and established his Technique there. For a time he spent alternate six-month periods in Britain and America.

By 1925 he had settled back in London, and set up a school to teach his Technique to children. This school carried on until 1934 when it moved to Bexley in Kent.

THE ALEXANDER TECHNIQUE TRAINING COURSE

By the time Alexander had reached the age of sixty he was under pressure from many quarters to set up a training school for teachers in case he died before leaving an heir to carry on his work. In 1931 he set up the first Alexander Technique Training Course in his home at Ashley Place. He went on teaching privately as well as training teachers until his death in October 1955.

Since his death the Technique has become famous throughout the world as more and more people turn to it in the hope of finding a solution to problems when all else has failed.

Chapter 2

THE QUEST BEGINS

All inquiry and learning is but recollection.

SOCRATES

It is important to remember that it was Alexander's overriding passion for the theatre that gave him the unswerving determination to see his task through in spite of the many setbacks along the way.

The story that follows is a tale of exploration, an important voyage of discovery of one man into himself and into the workings of the whole of mankind. It is a complex journey and it may take at least two or three readings of this chapter to become acquainted with Alexander's way of thinking and the basic principles upon which his Technique is based.

All these principles are explained in detail throughout the rest of the book, so I suggest you might like to re-read this chapter again at the end.

If you will do what I did, you will be able to do what I do.
Frederick Matthias Alexander

After Alexander's conversation with his doctor he was left with only two leads: One was his observation that the hoarseness in his voice appeared when he was reciting; and the second was that when he rested his voice, or was confined to ordinary talking, the hoarseness disappeared.

The journey had begun. He began to observe himself minutely in the mirror, first while he was speaking in an ordinary voice, and then while he was reciting some Shakespeare. He repeated the experiment many times and found that while he was merely speaking he noticed nothing unusual, but when he was reciting he saw that three things were happening:

1. He tended to pull back his head onto the spine.
2. He depressed his larynx (the area of the throat containing the vocal cords).
3. He began to suck in breath through the mouth in a way that produced a gasping sound.

After noting these tendencies he watched himself again during ordinary speech and found he was doing exactly the same three actions, but to a lesser degree, which was why he had not perceived them before. When he discovered this marked difference between what he did in ordinary speaking and what he did in reciting, he realized he had a definite clue which might explain things, and thus he was encouraged to explore further.

The next step was to find a way to prevent or change these damaging tendencies, and here he found himself in a maze. He asked himself the following questions:

1. Was it the sucking in of the breath that caused the pulling back of the head and the depressing of the larynx?
   or
2. Was it the pulling back of the head that caused the depressing of the larynx and the sucking in of breath?
   or
3. Was it the depressing of the larynx that caused the sucking in of the breath and the pulling back of the head?

He was unable to answer these questions at first, so he went on patiently experimenting in front of the mirror. After some months he realized that he was unable directly to prevent the sucking in of air or the depression of the larynx, but that he could to some extent prevent the pulling back of the head. This led to an even more important discovery, namely, that when he did succeed in preventing the pulling back of his head, this indirectly lessened the sucking in of air and eased the pressure on the larynx.

At this point he wrote in his journal:

The importance of this discovery cannot be over-estimated, for through it I was led on to the further discovery of the primary control of the working of all the mechanisms of the human organism, and this marked the first important stage of my investigation.

It is important here to take a break from the story to clarify what Alexander meant by 'the primary control'.

THE PRIMARY CONTROL

The 'Primary Control' acts as the main organizer of the body. It governs the working of all our mechanisms and so renders the control of our complex human organism comparatively simple. It is the dynamic relationship between our head and the rest of our body, and is often referred to as 'the head–neck–back relationship'. It is important to point out that this relationship is not one of position, but one of freedom of each to the other.

When the Primary Control is interfered with it can interfere with other reflexes throughout the body and cause a lack of co-ordination and balance. This can be seen in horses. When a rider wishes to stop the horse, he or she pulls the horse's head back with the reins. The animal immediately loses its co-ordination and soon comes to a standstill. It can also be demonstrated on a pet cat: if the cat's head is gently tipped in a backward direction the cat cannot function properly until it re-establishes control over its head, neck and back in relation to each other.

After his initial discovery of the 'Primary Control', Alexander noted further that when he was able to prevent the misuse of his head and larynx, the hoarseness in his voice decreased accordingly. When he was later examined by the medical profession, there was a considerable improvement in the condition of his vocal cords and larynx. This confirmed his suspicion that the way he used himself had a marked effect on the functioning of his respiration and voice. (Alexander was extremely precise in the words and phrases he used to describe his new discoveries. For example, a term like 'using himself', as above, may sound strange, but it is more correct than 'using his body', since he was talking about using his whole self and not just his body.)

So the second major observation was:

THE WAY IN WHICH HE USED HIMSELF DIRECTLY
AFFECTED HIS PERFORMANCE.

After giving the matter some thought, he concluded that if he put his head even further forward he might influence the functioning of his voice still more as a way of eliminating the hoarseness altogether. So he proceeded to 'put' his head forward. He found, however, that past a certain point he tended once again to pull his head down as well as forward, which in turn had the same damaging effect on his vocal and respiratory organs.

Alexander continued to experiment over a long period of time, and this led him to see that by using his head and neck in this way there was also a tendency to lift his chest and shorten his whole stature. This observation had far-reaching implications as we shall presently see.

So the next important observation was:

PULLING BACK HIS HEAD AFFECTED HIS WHOLE STRUCTURE.

Alexander experimented still further and noticed that his tendency to lift the chest also caused him to increase the arch of his spine, which in turn narrowed his back. This led him to the conclusion that:

THE MISUSE HE HAD NOTICED WAS NOT JUST OF SPECIFIC PARTS (AS AT FIRST PRESUMED) BUT OF HIS WHOLE BEING.

He then examined the effect that shortening and lengthening had on his voice. He found that the best results (that is, when he was least hoarse) happened when he lengthened his stature. In trying to do this, however, he found that he shortened more often than he lengthened. Looking for an explanation for this he saw that he had a tendency to pull his head down as well as back. Thus he realized that in order to maintain a lengthened structure:

HE MUST PUT HIS HEAD FORWARD AND UP.

Alexander believed he had finally solved his problem, but this was not yet the case. When it came to reciting, while trying to put his head forward and up, he noticed that he was still lifting his chest, arching his spine and narrowing his back. This made him suspect that what he *thought* he was doing, and what he was actually doing, were two different things.

At this stage in the proceedings he brought in two other mirrors, one on each side of the original. With their aid he could see that his suspicions were justified, and that when he attempted to maintain a lengthening in stature and speak at the same time, he actually pulled his head back (and not forward as he had intended). He had just stumbled upon what he later called faulty sensory perception.

FAULTY SENSORY PERCEPTION

In simple terms this means that the sensory feedback system that informs us where we are in space in relation to the earth may sometimes be untrustworthy. This also applies to the relationship of one part of our body to another. As in Alexander's case, what we *feel* we are doing may in fact be the opposite of what we are actually doing. This is probably the biggest pitfall when learning the Technique and I will come back to this subject later.

Alexander was very disturbed at this point. Even though he had located the cause of his problem, and believed he had found the remedy, he was unable to make use of it because he could not carry out the actions he had intended. He carefully reviewed the situation, and decided there was nothing for it but to persevere.

He continued experimenting on himself month after month with both successes and failures. He began to notice a great deal of undue muscle tension, particularly in his legs, feet and toes. His toes were contracted and bent downwards in such a way as made his feet unduly arched and threw the weight of his body onto the outside of his feet. Naturally this adversely affected his whole balance. Alexander was convinced that the abnormal amount of muscle tension in his legs and feet was indirectly associated with the loss of his voice.

DIRECTION

It slowly dawned on Alexander that his efforts up until now had been misdirected, and this led him to ask: 'What is this direction upon which I have been depending?' He had to admit that he had never thought about how he directed himself but had used himself in a way that felt natural to him.

He stopped at this point to examine all the information he had acquired so far. The particular issues he had noted were:

1. that the pulling of his head back and down when he felt

that he was putting it forward and up was proof that the movement of the particular parts concerned was being misdirected and that this misdirection was connected with his untrustworthy feelings;

2. that this misdirection was unconscious and together with the associated untrustworthy feeling, was part and parcel of his habitual use of himself;

3. that this unconscious misdirection leading to a wrong habitual use of himself, including in particular the incorrect use of his head and neck, came into play as the result of a decision to use his voice. In other words this misdirection was an instinctive response to the stimulus to use his voice.

The next step was to discover which direction would be necessary to bring about a new and improved use of the head and neck, therefore indirectly influencing the larynx, the breathing and other mechanisms of the body.

Alexander saw that if he was ever to react satisfactorily when using his voice, he must replace his old instinctive (unreasoned) habits by a new, conscious (reasoned) use of himself. While reciting he started consciously to 'direct' himself in such a way as to correct his old inappropriate habits. He was immediately confronted by a series of startling and unexpected experiences:

1. He found no clear dividing-line between reasoned and unreasoned directions.

2. He was successful in using himself in a new improved way until the point of actually speaking, when he reverted to his old habitual use.

3. As soon as he attempted to gain an end (that is, reciting), his unconscious habits dominated his reasoned directions (orders).

Alexander was extremely disappointed at these findings. Although he was making many discoveries from his experiments, he seemed to be unable to change the way in which he used himself while reciting. In exasperation he gave up trying to 'do' anything to gain his end, and at last saw that if he was ever to control his instinctive unconscious habits, he must at first refuse to 'do' anything immediately in response to the stimulus of speaking. He called this 'inhibition'.

INHIBITION

He realized that by giving up and not trying to do anything, and by merely thinking of his direction, he had achieved what he had been trying to do for several years. In other words simply by thinking of his head going forward and upwards he prevented the pulling back of the head, which in turn lengthened his stature and produced a beneficial effect on his larynx and vocal cords.

At this point he wrote:

> After I had worked on this plan for a considerable time, I became free from my tendency to revert to my wrong habitual use in reciting, and the marked effect of this upon my functioning convinced me that I was at last on the right track, for once free from this tendency, I also became free from the throat and vocal trouble and from the respiratory and nasal difficulties with which I had been beset from birth.

So, as so often happens, Alexander had stumbled almost accidentally on some crucial information about the functioning of the body, and how we interfere with many of our processes without even realizing we are doing so. When Alexander first noticed that he interfered with his body reflexes by pulling his head back and down, he thought this was merely a personal idiosyncrasy. Later, through teaching others, he realized that in fact this interference was practically universal to the whole human race.

Chapter 3

WHY DO WE NEED THE ALEXANDER TECHNIQUE?

You translate everything, whether physical or mental or spiritual, into muscular tension.

FREDERICK MATTHIAS ALEXANDER

The Alexander Technique is a very simple yet profound way of becoming more aware of the balance, posture and co-ordination of our bodies as we perform our numerous everyday activities. This subsequently allows us to be more aware of the excessive muscular tension that most of us unknowingly hold within our bodies. These undetected tensions gradually build up over many years until later on in life they result in stiffness, pain and even deformities, which we accept as an inevitable part of old age.

At first it is difficult to comprehend that the deterioration we take for granted is neither normal nor inevitable. And because we are led to believe that so many of our aches and pains are caused by general wear and tear, we do little to find a remedy for them. We ignore the discomfort without question, and when the doctor responds with, 'What do you expect at your age?', this merely confirms what we think already.

Many of our ailments are directly caused or exacerbated by bad posture, and can be avoided if we use our bodies in a co-ordinated way throughout our life. Pain is nature's last resort; its way of informing us that something is wrong. Yet there are many other signals earlier on, which we tend to ignore or are unaware of. And even when we are in a great deal of pain, instead of listening to what our body is trying to tell us, we tend to block out the symptoms with a variety of pain-killing drugs. (Obviously pain-killing drugs have their place, but in our culture they are generally over-prescribed.)

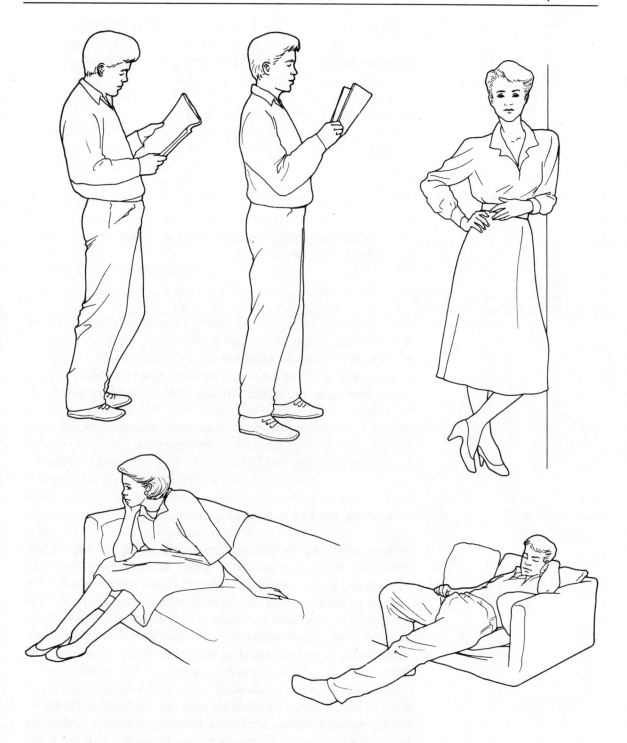

Fig. 1 The way in which we stand or sit can put many muscles under stress without us realizing it.

We need to ask ourselves what it is that causes so much physical suffering in our modern civilization. We might then gain an insight into how we could sit, stand or move in a less stressful way, in order to relieve our aches and pains.

Good posture is rare. The way in which we hold our bodies is the result of an accumulation of life's past experiences – physical, emotional and mental. We become trapped in certain postures, not realizing that the rigid shape we have acquired is unnatural or that it can lead to ill-health in the future. An example of this is depression. It is easy to see how this mental disorder could be connected to the way people collapse down into themselves; whereas if they were to stand or sit in a more upright or poised manner they would tend to suffer less from depression.

REASONS WHY OUR POSTURE CHANGES WITH AGE

- the many hours of sitting at school;
- lack of exercise in later years;
- our 'fear reflex' that is constantly being stimulated;
- the speed with which we often have to accomplish our tasks;
- the goal-oriented attitude that we are taught as children;
- a distinct lack of interest in the present;
- the development of habits, both physical and mental.

The many hours of sitting at school

In his early years a child moves freely and naturally. If you observe the posture of a four-year-old child and then of a sixteen-year-old adolescent you will find very obvious and startling differences. The four-year-old will be more upright in a natural and effortless way, whereas the sixteen-year-old will be much more slumped, and in order to keep himself erect while standing or sitting will invariably pull in the lower back. This will cause a shortening of the whole structure.

This process begins within a few months of starting school. Any primary school teacher will tell you that young children do not want to sit still, yet because of the high ratio of children to teachers it is the only way to maintain order in the classroom. Sitting for a short while is fine, especially when it

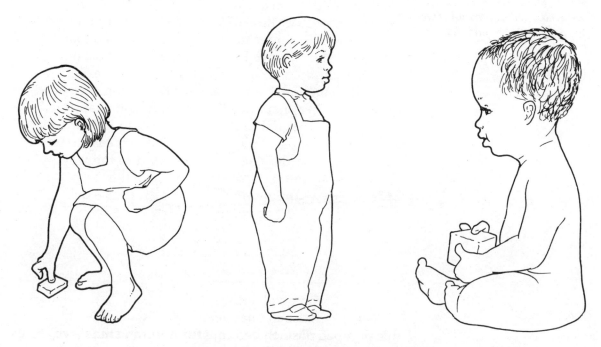

Fig. 2 The poise and grace of movement that we have as children.

is the child's free choice, but the number of hours that children have to sit increases with age until in the early teens a child can sit for as many as ten hours a day when homework and television are taken into consideration. This is harmful on two accounts:

(a) holding the body still for any length of time causes the tiring and consequently tensing of numerous muscles; and
(b) the design of chairs in general does not take into account the mechanics of the human structure. The natural tendency for everyone is to collapse down into a slumped position while sitting in chairs or sofas.

It is also important to realize that the spine is under greater pressure when sitting than in almost any other position.

If you observe children carefully, you will notice they sink down into themselves each time their minds start to wander. Because of the exorbitant number of hours we spend sitting,

Fig. 3 Many years of hunching over school work can seriously affect our posture and breathing later in life.

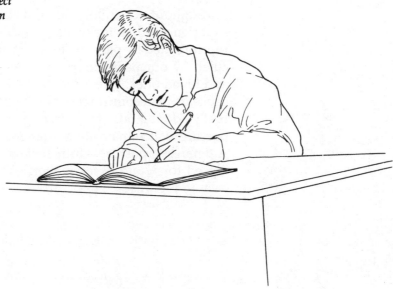

this slumped position becomes the norm and thus crystallizes into our habitual way of being.

An average child who starts school at the age of five and leaves at the age of eighteen will probably have sat for more than forty thousand hours during that time; that is, over half their waking life.

Lack of exercise in later years

This lack of movement because of prolonged sitting does not stop once we leave school. I asked a total of four hundred people from all walks of life: 'What is the total number of hours you spend sitting down during an average day?' Answers ranged from four to a staggering fourteen hours, the average being about nine hours.

It is because many of us use so few of our muscles to their maximum capacity that we slowly begin to lose much of our flexibility until we end up in old age scarcely able to move. Yet even at the age of eighty-five Alexander could balance perfectly on one leg while he swung the other leg over the back of a chair three feet in height, a feat that most people in their thirties would find difficult.

Our fear reflex that is constantly being stimulated

Throughout our childhood, and also in adult life we all have experiences that make us withdraw. These include being reprimanded by parents, teachers and employers, being ridiculed by our peer group, and being rejected by our friends and loved ones. These incidents, if frequently repeated, can cause us to become excessively introverted and we will eventually adopt a posture reflecting our defensive attitude. This posture will remain long after the initial cause has ceased. A defensive posture – hunched or rounded shoulders, a collapsed torso and excessive tension in the neck muscles – is easy to identify.

The speed with which we often have to accomplish our tasks

We often have to accomplish many of our activities in a set time, far more than previous generations did. This will certainly lead to anxiety and tension, and if constantly repeated will cause us to adopt certain postures in response.

The goal-oriented attitude that we are taught as children

Alexander talked at length on the subject of 'goal orientation'. He referred to civilized man as a race of end-gainers. What he meant by this was that we are often more interested in achieving an end than experiencing the means whereby we reach that end. Because of this, our posture and co-ordination can be severely affected in the process of performing even the simplest tasks. It is almost unbelievable how much tremendous force intelligent human beings can employ throughout their whole bodies while performing such a simple action as standing up, simply because they are more interested in the end result than in how they should perform such an activity. If unchecked this will cause postural difficulties in later life.

A distinct lack of interest in the present

A lack of interest in the present is mainly brought on by the habitual way in which we are constantly looking to the future.

We are encouraged by society always to want more, always to look to the future which promises to be even more fulfilling. For example, for months and months before Christmas we are bombarded with advertisements for Christmas, and then on Boxing Day enticements for the summer holidays begin. Because of this lack of interest in the present our posture can change drastically over the year without our even noticing, until one day we catch sight of ourselves sideways-on in a mirror or on video.

The development of habits, both physical and mental

We all form habits, both of body and mind, most of which are below our level of consciousness. Our habits feel comfortable to us and are therefore difficult to change since everything else feels strange. But these habits can put our whole organism out of balance and soon we start to resume rigid positions, and become fixed in one posture or another.

Posture is an ever-changing process, depending on where we are in space. It could be said that 'bad posture' is a posture that is fixed in one place, and that 'good posture' is a posture that is always varying with different moods and movements of the body.

The effects of a rigid posture can be:

SHALLOW BREATHING – This will of course affect the whole system as oxygen is needed by every organ in the body.

OVER-TIREDNESS – The constant effort needed to keep a particular posture drains us of our energy which could be used to do the things we enjoy.

STRESS – Our whole system will be under constant tension which will eventually develop into pain.

DEPRESSION – It is well known that many people who suffer from depression have a very pronounced slumped posture.

It is important at this stage to note that better posture is only a by-product of practising the Alexander Technique and not, as most people think, the end in itself. By freeing muscular tension in the body, our postural muscles have a chance to work again thus restoring the natural posture and ease of movement we lost in childhood.

> Heaven lies about us in our infancy!
> Shades of the prison-house begin to close ·
> Upon the growing boy.
> William Wordsworth

Thus from about the age of five or six it is a downhill course, and by the age of nine or ten the process is well advanced. A child psychologist can tell whether a child is stressed simply by the way it holds its body. The child's defensive posture against a hostile world becomes frozen in time and the seeds of future ill-health are already sown. This is then seen in the adult – as an arched back or hunched shoulders. Many diseases and common ailments are caused or made worse by the tensions we unconsciously hold within us.

The cost of misusing our bodies is great not only to ourselves personally, but also to the community. Annual losses in productivity through back pain alone run into thousands of millions of pounds, and statistics and common sense tell us that our National Health Service is unable to meet the increasing demands made upon it. Many doctors work more than a hundred hours each week, which obviously places them under considerable stress and puts patients' lives at risk. Clearly some serious re-thinking is required, but unfortunately common sense seems to be lacking in so many areas of our lives. If you arrived home one day to find water dripping through the ceiling, you would not just paper over the wet patch; you would first find the reason for the leak to prevent the problem getting worse. Why is it, then, that when it comes to our health we only look at symptoms and rarely investigate the fundamental causes of so many of our illnesses?

The answer is that we simply do not know where to start, and this is where the Alexander Technique comes in.

Chapter 4

WHAT IS THE ALEXANDER TECHNIQUE?

Every man, woman and child holds the possibility of physical perfection; it rests with each one of us to attain it by personal understanding and effort.

FREDERICK MATTHIAS ALEXANDER

The Alexander Technique will help you to:

- move through life with greater ease;
- become more aware of yourself: physically, mentally and emotionally;
- prevent unnecessary wear and tear on your body;
- detect excessive muscular tension in yourself, and teach you how to let go of this unwanted tension;
- stop wasting your energy and find new ways of moving more efficiently, thus avoiding fatigue at the end of the day;
- recognize your patterns of behaviour, and change them if you so wish;
- become more conscious of your habitual ways of performing actions, thus allowing you the choice to make more appropriate decisions;
- rediscover the grace of movement you once had as a child;
- be truly free.

MOVING THROUGH LIFE WITH GREATER EASE

By applying the principles set out later in this book, you will be able to release habitual tensions and thus move in a very different way. This will make many of your everyday activities easier and allow you to enjoy life more fully. This in turn will affect the people around you. Your new-found happiness may 'rub off' on to those you are close to. I often hear comments such as, 'Since my husband has had Alexander lessons he is a much nicer man to live with;' or, 'I feel much calmer and more relaxed since I have become involved in the Alexander Technique.'

In so many ways we make life more difficult than it really needs to be. We see it in others, but not so easily in ourselves. Life can soon become a joy, rather than the struggle so many of us make it.

BECOMING MORE AWARE OF YOURSELF: PHYSICALLY, EMOTIONALLY AND MENTALLY

This is the first step on the road to change. When you begin to become more aware of yourself you will be astounded at how much effort it used to take to perform very simple actions. A person can severely damage their back just by picking up a lightweight object from the floor. The main reason we do not notice the stress on our bodies is that it increases by such minute amounts each day. Eventually, as this tension accumulates, it begins to interfere with the body's natural co-ordination and reflexes.

Our body, mind and emotions are all interconnected; and the way in which we move will in turn affect our mental and emotional well-being. Similarly the way in which we feel or think will influence the way in which we undertake our daily activities. In this way a vicious cycle is created which reduces our capacity to enjoy life.

PREVENTING UNNECESSARY WEAR AND TEAR ON YOUR BODY

By moving in a badly co-ordinated manner, the muscular and skeletal systems come under constant strain. Last year, for example, a newspaper reported that an American woman arrived at Heathrow Airport from New York and hired a car with a manual gearbox. She had only driven automatic vehicles back in her own country, and had no idea how to change gear. Consequently she drove a hundred and twenty miles to Bristol in first gear! She then complained to the rental company that the car didn't go very fast and was extremely noisy.

Obviously, because she was not using the car correctly, both the engine and gearbox were under enormous strain and probably suffered permanent damage.

In the same way, if we do not use ourselves as nature intended (and so many people today do not), we may unknowingly be inflicting irreversible damage that will manifest later on in life. It is worth remembering that you can always exchange your car when it wears out, but you cannot exchange your body for a new one.

DETECTING AND RELEASING EXCESSIVE MUSCULAR TENSION

As you gradually become aware of yourself, you will begin to notice the muscular tensions I have mentioned. Certain muscles become more and more tense while others become over relaxed. This process takes place over many years and will eventually affect the physiological structure of the muscles; in fact they diminish in size, and this is one of the main reasons why older people seem to shrink.

Most of us are completely ignorant of the effect this process has on our bodies, until we experience a pain. As our body starts to break down we visit the doctor, hoping for answers she/he is unable to give. We rarely ask ourselves: 'What am I doing to myself that could be causing this pain?'

If we could find the answer to this question, we would stop doing it and the pain would ease naturally and soon disappear. However, because the tensions build up gradually over many years the cause is often hard to detect. We become so used to certain stress levels in the body that we accept them as part of ourselves.

Letting go of these stresses is a relatively simple procedure once we have recognized the reason for them.

CONSERVING ENERGY BY FINDING NEW WAYS OF MOVING

The Alexander Technique will help you to stop and think before proceeding with your actions. This will allow you to do any activity with much greater efficiency of movement; in other words, to perform tasks with much less effort. This in turn will leave you with more energy to do the things you want to do. You will experience more vitality and this will enhance your life. Young children seem to have endless reserves of energy. This is because they use their bodies in a co-ordinated way and do not waste energy as most adults do.

RECOGNIZING AND CHANGING YOUR PATTERNS OF BEHAVIOUR

As we have said, throughout life we all develop physical, mental and emotional patterns of behaviour. Other people are often more aware of them than we are ourselves. We will respond to a given stimulus in a set way, irrespective of whether or not it is appropriate to the situation. As many of these patterns are below our level of consciousness, we will repeat them again and again without realizing what we are doing.

The Alexander Technique will enable you to perceive these habitual behavioural tendencies in order to change them if they are having a detrimental effect on your well-being. The implications are far-reaching because you will have more freedom of choice. You will be able to behave in an appropriate way in any situation that life presents, thus avoiding stress or illness later on.

RECOGNIZING AND CHANGING YOUR HABITUAL WAYS OF PERFORMING ACTIONS

Many of us, in Western civilization, use our bodies in a clumsy and awkward manner. We often perform our actions in a stereotyped way, and this habit feels 'right' to us, regardless of the strain it puts on our structure. In this way, by placing excessive demands on ourselves, serious damage may be caused to our bodies. Many thousands of people suffer from a prolapsed intervertebral disc (more commonly known as a slipped disc). This is often caused by constant repetition of bending down in such a way that the spine is put under strain. The pressure is so great that the intervertebral disc is caught in a vice between the two adjacent vertebrae (*see* Chapter 14: Give Your Back a Rest).

By simply stopping for a moment to find the easiest way of performing any action, we not only avoid inflicting an unnecessary burden upon ourselves, but we may also save ourselves a great deal of time in the long run. Old proverbs such as 'look before you leap' or 'more haste, less speed' are very appropriate in this fast-moving world in which we now find ourselves.

RECREATING THE GRACE OF MOVEMENT YOU HAD AS A CHILD

The Alexander Technique is not so much a process of learning, but more a way of remembering what we have long since forgotten. It could be defined as a process of unlearning or re-education of the entire psycho-physical functioning of the human being.

Alexander himself often said that if you stop doing what is wrong, then the right thing will happen automatically. In other words, when we stop interfering with the natural reflexes and co-ordination of the body, then the body will perform with optimum efficiency and with greater ease of movement.

No matter what our age, we can regain some of that graceful, poised way of being that we see so clearly in young children, which is still latent in each and every one of use. I have taught pupils up to the age of eighty-four who have benefited from a course of lessons. Even very elderly people are able to move more freely and can do far more without becoming fatigued.

To start moving in these new ways, we need to become aware of the extent to which we interfere with many of our body's natural processes, including the respiratory, nervous and circulatory systems. Our children can in fact be our greatest teachers. Spending a few moments watching a child of three or four playing on the beach or in the park can teach us much about the way our bodies were originally designed to be used. This is quite different from the way to which we become accustomed in our later years.

Most people report a feeling of lightness and a greater sense of well-being even after just one or two Alexander lessons. At first this sensation is only temporary, but with further lessons tends to become permanent.

BECOMING FREE

As a result of Alexander's observations, both about himself and others, he became more and more convinced that the body, the mind, the emotions and the spirit are inseparable, and that if any one of these is misused the other three will be affected.

It is not difficult to see that the way we think influences the way we feel, and that this in turn affects our general performance in life. Our successes and our apparent failures lead us to think of ourselves in a certain way. Equally, when we learn to develop a new freedom in the way we move, we will also be able to free our thoughts from preconceived ideas and fixed prejudices and will be able to think and feel differently about many issues in our lives. This process will ultimately guide us to the freedom of our spirit, bringing us a sense of happiness and fulfilment which we may not have enjoyed since childhood.

Throughout history men and women have given their lives for the freedom of family or country, yet few realize that they are trapped by the habitual way they think, and are imprisoned by the growing pressures daily inflicted upon them. This is not to say we should live outside the rules we have set for ourselves, but rather than we should consciously choose not to react in a way that is detrimental to ourselves or to those around us.

The actual practice of the Alexander Technique is set down clearly and simply in the following chapters of this book, but it is useful at this stage to see what it does and does not offer.

THE ALEXANDER TECHNIQUE IS:

- a way of understanding how the body is naturally designed to work;
- a method of heightening our awareness, both of ourselves and the world around us;
- a re-education of how to use the body in such a way that our psycho-physical equilibrium can be restored;
- a process which can help us to recognize the interference that we ourselves inflict upon the body's natural functions;
- a way to use our thinking capacity to bring about a desired change so that we may go about our daily activities in a more co-ordinated fashion;
- a way of becoming more aware on many levels;
- a technique that you can practise on your own, to help you move in a way that carries the minimum amount of tension

at any given time. (*Note*: obviously we need a certain amount of tension to function; the trouble is we often over-do it.)

THE ALEXANDER TECHNIQUE IS NOT:

- a therapy;
- a form of treatment of any kind;
- anything to do with massage, or the like;
- a form of healing – although the body's natural healing processes may well be activated;
- an exercise programme in any shape or form;
- manipulation;
- a complementary medicine, such as homoeopathy, acupuncture or osteopathy. You do not have to be ill or have something wrong with you to gain benefit from the Technique. It just so happens that many of us only start to look at the way we live in times of crisis. (It is worth reminding ourselves that prevention is better than cure.)

In short, the Alexander Technique is something we learn in order to help ourselves, rather than a treatment whereby a doctor or therapist 'does something' to the patient.

Chapter 5

How Alexander's Discovery is Relevant Today

Men do more things through habit than through reason.

OLD PROVERB

THE PRESSURES OF EVERYDAY LIVING

In this chapter I hope to make clear how Alexander's discovery can be of use to us in our everyday lives. As you will remember, his vocal problems stemmed from unnecessary muscle tension which occurred when he reacted to the stimulus of reciting. Today we are bombarded with stimuli from all quarters because the world about us moves at such a fast pace. Our automatic reflex system is under constant pressure to keep up with the ever-growing pace of life and for this reason we start to function in unconscious, habitual ways.

We rarely stop to think whether there may be an easier or more appropriate way of going about even the simplest tasks and our bodies begin to build up severe tensions, completely unnoticed until we start to feel pain. For example, there is the learner driver who clenches the steering wheel with such a strong grip that his hands ache afterwards. He is unaware of this completely unnecessary and inappropriate overactivity of the muscular system. Because of the enormous demands put on us by modern-day living, we build up stress that for the most part goes unnoticed and therefore unchecked. We have made our lives far more complex than they really need to be. Just consider for a moment how we go about a simple task like shopping. We take our car to the shops, drive around for ten minutes looking for a parking space, and then watch in frustration as someone takes the space we have been waiting for. When we eventually find a space, we usually only have a certain length of time to do the shopping, so if anything delays us we have to rush back to our car before we get a parking ticket. Similarly, think about getting the children to school on time. We have all seen exhausted parents standing outside the school in the morning. Most children have a completely different sense of time from adults, so parents have constantly to nag their children to be punctual, and this is a strain on all concerned.

There are countless situations in everyday life that cause us to be stressed. This stress is then transmitted into muscular tension and if left unchecked can go on to contribute to one of the numerous stress-related illnesses listed below:

- Hypertension (commonly known as high blood pressure);
- Coronary thrombosis (one of the major causes of death in Western civilization);
- Gastro-intestinal conditions (stomach ulcers are well known as a stress-related illness);
- Headaches;
- Migraine (more than six million people suffer from migraine in England alone);
- Insomnia;
- Arthritis;
- Backache.

Hypertension is raised blood pressure, it can rise to a point where there is a risk of cardiac damage or stroke. The cause of high blood pressure is still obscure; at present it is generally believed to occur when the smaller arteries go into spasm. It is thought that this spasm is produced by adrenaline, and that adrenaline is produced by emotional, mental or physical strain.

Experiments have been carried out in laboratories by scientists and medical practitioners, including Professor Frank Pierce Jones, Doctor Wilfred Barlow and Chris Stevens (physicist). They report a significant drop in blood pressure in patients prone to hypertension, even after attending only a few Alexander lessons. This is obviously an attractive alternative to the many drugs available today because not only do Alexander lessons produce no adverse side affects but they may actually be cheaper than many of the expensive hypotensive drugs. It is interesting to note that in 1989 over £118,000,000 was spent by British people on pain-killing drugs.

Coronary Thrombosis, more commonly known as a heart attack, is caused by a narrowing of a major branch of one of the coronary arteries. It could be that this narrowing is caused by the over-tensing of the muscles that surround this particular artery. In his book *The Alexander Principle*, Doctor Wilfred Barlow reports:

I see a good number of people who have had a coronary thrombosis. I have never yet seen a case in which the upper chest was not markedly raised and over-contracted. I regard it as essential that such patients should be taught to release their chest tension and to do so in a way that is accompanied by an improvement in their general use.

So it is clear that the disease which claims nearly two hundred thousand deaths each year in England alone is exacerbated as a result of a build-up of tension, caused by the stress of everyday life.

Gastro-intestinal conditions figure high on the list of stress-related disorders. An example of this is the stomach ulcer, an extremely painful condition often associated with high-pressure occupations which subject people to constant undue strain. An ulcer, or a similar ailment, will often develop within a short period as a signal to slow down.

One of the main aims of the Technique is to help us take our time, and by doing so accomplish far more. Hence the saying: 'More haste, less speed.'

Tension Headaches are extremely common today, usually caused by over-tightening of the neck and shoulder muscles (the sterno-mastoid and the trapezius). In my experience Alexander pupils who suffer from headaches say that the pain soon becomes less intense, and the headaches less frequent. It is also my experience that if a pupil comes to me with a headache, once they are able to relax the appropriate muscles the pain has often gone by the end of the lesson.

Migraine is becoming more and more common, with over six million sufferers in Britain. While this condition is often related to a hormonal imbalance and is more common in women than in men, it is rare to find someone who cannot be helped by learning to release some of the tension that they hold around the neck, head, shoulders and face. The medical profession states that although migraines are due to a chemical imbalance they can be provoked or made worse by stressful conditions such as anxiety, loud noises, physical and mental fatigue, emotional upset, and depression.

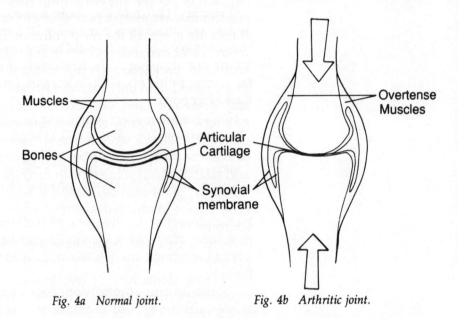

Fig. 4a   *Normal joint.*   Fig. 4b   *Arthritic joint.*

Insomnia is often caused by anxiety in some form. People who suffer from this condition often have an over-active mind – they worry about details of the day and consequently become more annoyed when they cannot sleep. By practising the Alexander Technique they can release much of the tension that has built up over the years and this in turn helps them to feel calmer and able to sleep better, thus breaking the cycle.
Osteo Arthritis is the term applied to the chronic degeneration and ultimate deformity of the bones that make up a joint. This could be caused by a permanent over-tightening of the muscles that connect the two bones involved (*see* figures 4a and 4b).

As you can see from Fig. 4b, the muscles shorten to such an extent that the two connecting bones start to rub against each other and begin to wear down. It is easy to imagine how much tension it takes to erode a substance as hard as bone. It is important to note, however, that once the muscle is able to lengthen again, the bones return to their original position (*see* Fig. 4a) and, because bone is living tissue, it will repair itself again. Thus arthritis sufferers often experience relief once they begin to become aware of and release the muscle tension they have unconsciously been holding.

After a series of case studies, Doctor Barlow (a consultant rheumatologist and teacher of the Alexander Technique) reported to the Royal Society of Medicine that over ninety-five per cent of people suffering from rheumatoid arthritis incurred the disease after a period of stress.

Backache is one of the most common illnesses in our society today. Over two million people in England alone are often off work with backache each year (often that is over half a million every week). This only includes Britain's actual working force, and does not take into account children, senior citizens, mothers with young children, the unemployed, and many others who do not work for one reason or another. Over eight per cent of the adult population experiences severe lower back and sciatic pain at some time in their lives.

Because of the number of people who are afflicted with backache I have dedicated a whole chapter to the subject (*see* Chapter 14).

As you can see from these few examples the growing pressures of living in the twentieth century place ever-increasing demands on our bodies and minds. I always remember a friend saying to me, 'Whoever wins the rat-race is still a rat!'

It is obvious that most of us cannot change our life styles: the children still have to be taken to school on time, the bills still have to be paid, and we still need to perform tasks that are potentially stressful. However, we can choose not to react to the ever-present stimuli in a way that is detrimental to our well-being. You can start to do this by practising the following:

Give yourself plenty of time to get where you are going. Try not to leave things until the last minute, especially when being late is bound to cause tension.

Avoid deadlines whenever possible. Don't tie yourself down to specific times when more general ones will do. For example, say 'I will meet you between 8.30 and 9.00' rather than 'I will see you at 8.45.'

Allow time for yourself. Don't run yourself down. Set aside some time each day for the things you really enjoy doing. Try to listen to your body, for there are many signs our body gives us before illness occurs. It is worth remembering: *Human beings say that time passes away. But time says that it is the human beings that pass away.*

Live each day to the full. Concern yourself with the present; yesterday cannot be changed and tomorrow has not yet come.

The only time we ever have is today. Thomas Carlyle once wrote:

> Our main business is not to see what lies dimly at a distance, but to do what lies clearly at hand.

Most of the problems to our life stem from the simple fact that we are very rarely totally present while we perform our tasks; we are usually thinking about something else completely. Alexander called this 'the mind-wandering habit'. It is impossible to put the Technique into practice until we become attentive to each action we perform. In this connection I often refer to a poem written by the famous Indian dramatist, Kalidasa:

> *Salutation to the Dawn*
> Look to this day!
> For it is life, the very life of life.
> In its brief course
> Lie all the verities and realities of your existence:
>   The bliss of growth
>   The glory of action
>   The splendour of achievement,
> For yesterday is but a dream
> And tomorrow is only a vision,
> But today well lived makes yesterday a dream of happiness
> And every tomorrow a vision of hope.
> Look well, therefore, to this day!
> Such is the salutation to the dawn.

PREVENTION OF DISEASE

It is important to mention that although most people do not turn to the Alexander Technique until they are in pain, a healthy person can benefit enormously from practising this Technique. Not only will it result in a lightness of being and increased awareness, but will help to prevent permanently many of the problems already mentioned. With the growing pressures around us it is essential to find a practical way of being aware of, and thus able to let go of the many tensions we accumulate from day to day.

There are an increasing number of stress-management courses and relaxation classes available, yet we hardly every get to the root of what makes us stressed in the first place. In the Western world we have insurance policies to protect us from the external changes that may happen in our lives, yet we never consider protecting ourselves from the internal changes that result in so many ailments.

It is interesting that many years ago people in China only paid their doctor when they were well and not (as we do today) when they fell sick. As a result, there was a great incentive for the doctor to keep his patients well. We often fail to value our health until we become ill, so we ignore the signals our body is giving us. We do not realize that stiffness and inflexibility can nearly always be avoided if we use ourselves in a different way. The Alexander Technique helps to free us from the habits of a lifetime, bringing renewed flexibility and ease of movement.

Exercise

The first thing to do to reduce muscle tension is to **stop and do nothing** for at least a few minutes each day just to be with yourself. In this way you may begin to notice tension or muscular strain before it builds up and causes further physical problems. Just find ten minutes in your day to go off and be alone – it does not matter whether you sit or lie down. For this short time it is best not to have the radio or television on, or any other distraction.

Just practise being alone with your thoughts. In this way you will begin to bring your body to a state of stillness. At first the ten minutes will feel endless, but as you get used to this quiet space in your day the ten minutes will pass in no time at all.

It is hard to put aside all your responsibilities at first, but they will all be taken care of in due course – we often forget that to take care of *ourselves* is one of our most important responsibilities.

Chapter 6

HOW CAN WE BEGIN TO HELP OURSELVES?

Education is an admirable thing. But it is well to remember from time to time that nothing that is worth knowing can be taught.

OSCAR WILDE

It is essential to point out that this book is not a substitute for lessons in the Alexander Technique, in the same way as a 'teach-yourself-to-drive' book would not preclude the need for driving lessons. It should be used as a helpful guide prior to or in conjunction with actual Alexander lessons, whether individual or group sessions.

The main reason for this is that it is much easier for a person who is objective, and experienced in this field, to see clearly the 'misuse' of his or her pupil. Remember, it took Alexander many hours a day over several years to discover what caused him to lose his voice. Most of us have neither the time nor the patience to achieve what he did; nor is it necessary. He left behind enough clues to make the process of self-discovery far easier, but it is still advisable to have a guide, for the path has numerous pitfalls and obstacles along the way.

It is worth reiterating that we are not learning anything new; this is a process of unlearning. Once we stop doing what is causing the problem, the 'right thing' will automatically take its place.

AWARENESS AND OBSERVATION

Observation of ourselves and others is the first major step to becoming aware of how much we misuse our bodies in even the simplest of activities. It is much easier to see it in others at first, simply because you are more objective. When observing other people try to study the whole of them rather than specific parts, and ask yourself these following questions:

Is this person

(a) standing up straight?
(b) leaning forwards?
(c) leaning backwards?

If they are leaning forwards or backwards, where does the lean start from?

(a) from the ankles?
(b) from the hips?
(c) from the upper back or shoulders?

A side view may be the best way of seeing clearly the mis-shapen forms so many of us have. You will often notice two or more different tendencies with opposing forces: for example, someone may be leaning back from their waist while their head and shoulders are thrown forward from the upper part of the chest (*see* Fig. 6). It is also interesting to watch the differing postures that people adopt while they are sitting. If possible, notice the varying shapes that individuals adopt as life's internal and external pressures take their toll.

When you start to acquire a sense of the lack of poise in many of the people you see, begin to observe yourself to see whether you are doing the same thing. It is essential that you remain as objective as possible, and it helps to have a sense of humour! Alexander used to say, 'This work is all too serious to be taken seriously.'

If you do notice anything about yourself which you think could be improved, it is important not to try and bring about a change immediately. Anything you do will invariably cause an increase in tension, thus encouraging the habit to become more ingrained. Our human tendency is to bring about the end we desire straight away, but it is vital to use our reasoning and work out first what is causing the problem. In other words, we have to 'undo' something rather than 'do' something else, and this is easier said than done. This is when Alexander lessons can be invaluable; your teacher will spot immediately when tension in your body is being increased rather than decreased.

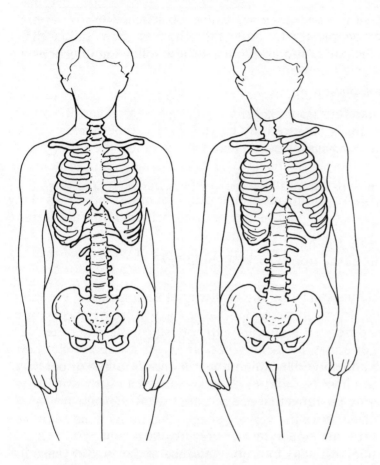

Fig. 5 Unbalanced posture can put a strain on our entire skeletal system as well as on all the internal organs.

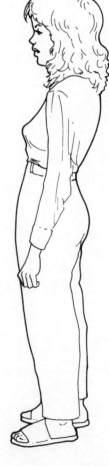

Fig. 6 A common standing position – the person is leaning back from their waist, while her head and shoulders are thrown forward.

STANDING

To become more aware of yourself while standing, ask the following questions:

1. Am I standing more on one leg than the other, or am I equally balanced on both of my legs? (Even if you are equally balanced, try moving over so that there is slightly more weight on one leg than the other, then reverse the process. Whichever position feels more comfortable will indicate your habit.)
2. Am I standing more on my heels or more on the balls of my feet? (This will help to indicate whether you are leaning backwards or forwards.)
3. Am I standing more on the outside or on the inside of my feet? (*Note*: this may be different for each foot; for example you may be standing on the outside of the left foot and on the inside of the right.)
4. Are my knees locked back with excess tension, or are they over-relaxed so that my knees are bent?

Any other aspects of standing will involve our sense of feeling which may be extremely unreliable, and it is therefore necessary to use either a mirror or a video camera to obtain accurate information.

If, by asking any of the previous questions, you begin to notice you have a habit of standing in an unbalanced way, it is helpful to exaggerate the tendency for a short while to get a sense of how much strain is caused throughout your whole structure. In other words, if you are inclined to stand more on your left leg and on the outside of your feet, then exaggerate this habit still further, so as to stand even more on to your left side and more on the outside of your feet. Within a few moments you will begin to get a sense of your whole structure being out of balance. This feeling is always with us to a certain extent, but we are unaware of it because our habit overrides our kinaesthetic sense (the sense that tells us where we are in space).

Simply by being conscious of the way we stand we will start to bring about a change that is desirable for our well-being.

Improving your standing position

Although Alexander did not advocate a correct way of standing, as this would encourage a new set of habits, he did leave behind a few useful suggestions to remember while standing:

1. The feet could be at approximately a 45-degree angle with about nine inches between them. This gives a more solid base on which to support the rest of the body.
2. When standing for long periods, it is helpful to place one foot slightly behind the other, with the weight of the body resting chiefly on the rear foot. This prevents sinking down into one hip which can affect the balance of the whole structure. This is particularly helpful to those of us who have a habit of standing more on one leg than the

3. The hips should be allowed to go back without altering the balance and without deliberately throwing the body forward. This helps to eliminate the almost universal tendency of pushing the pelvis forward when in a standing position.

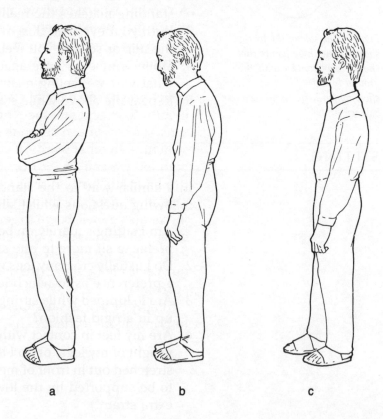

Fig. 7a Incorrect standing position – the lower back is hollowed, with the hips and stomach thrown forward, causing fatigue and bad internal pressures.

Fig. 7b Incorrect standing position – the shoulders are slumped again causing bad internal pressures and distorting the body.

Fig. 7c Improved standing position – see above.

a   b   c

4. There are three points on each foot which form a tripod. The first point is the heel, the second is the ball, and the third is situated at the beginning of the little toe. (*See* Figure 8.) It is well known by engineers that an object needs at least three points of contact to be stable; so if we are only standing on two of the three points we will be less balanced and consequently many more muscles will be tense trying to maintain the body's equilibrium. Next time your shoes wear out have a look at where they are worn down most as this will give a good indication about whether or not there is even pressure throughout the whole foot.

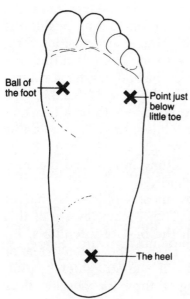

Ball of the foot

Point just below little toe

The heel

Fig. 8 The sole of the foot showing the three points that should be in contact with the ground in order to set up a tripod effect which helps us to keep our balance.

Exercise

Using a mirror:

1. Stand with your eyes closed, facing the mirror in a way that feels comfortable.
2. Open your eyes and see if your idea of how you were standing matches the reality.
3. With your eyes still closed, try to align yourself in front of the mirror so that you feel completely symmetrical.
4. Open your eyes once again, to see if what you see and what you are feeling match.
5. Repeat the above while standing sideways to the mirror.

SITTING

In a similar way to the standing exercise, you can ask the following questions whilst sitting:

1. Am I sitting squarely on both of my sitting bones, or do I prefer to sit more to one side?
2. Do I usually cross my legs while sitting, and if so do I have a preference as to which leg I cross?
3. Am I slumped while sitting, or do I have a tendency to sit up in a rigid fashion?
4. Are my feet in contact with the floor, thus supporting the weight of my legs, or do I have my legs under my chair or stretched out in front of me? (If this is so the legs will have to be supported by the lower back thus putting it under extra strain.)

5. Am I always inclined to use the back of the chair for support? (If this is so the postural muscles will slowly become under used.)

It is important to understand that no one sitting position is wrong. Our bodies can cope with almost any position for a short while: it is when we have a strong habit of sitting in a certain way that we put one part of the body under considerable tension for long periods of time. Because of this there are no shoulds or should nots but there needs to be a constant awareness of not becoming 'fixed' while sitting. Figures 9a and 9b show typical positions many people adopt when sitting; while Figure 9c shows a person sitting in a poised manner, neither slumping, not sitting up rigidly.

Fig. 9a   Sitting in a slumped way.

A common habit adopted by most children is that of slumping over the school desk. The teacher, aware of this undesirable tendency, and with the best of intentions, instructs the child to sit up straight. Then, either through fear or an eagerness to please, the child will over-straighten by pulling up the chest and contracting all the back muscles, thus

Fig. 9b   Sitting up too straight in a rigid fashion.

Fig. 9c   A nicely poised and balanced sitting position.

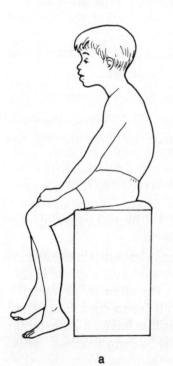

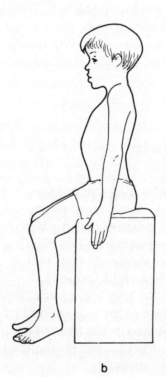

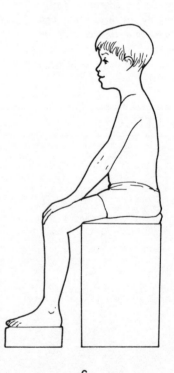

a   b   c

subsequently forming an over-exaggerated curve of the lumbar spine. Since the teacher can only see the child from the front he or she will not notice the accentuated arch in the lower back.

In this way, many children start to use their voluntary muscles to hold themselves in an upright position, and many years of repeating this habit will inevitably lead to chronic lower back pain. This is the most common type of pain. (The differences between voluntary and postural muscles are discussed in Chapter 12.)

Exercise

Here again a mirror can reveal whether we are suffering from faulty sensory perception:

1. Place your chair in front of a mirror and without looking into the mirror sit in your usual fashion.
2. Then look at your reflection to see if your idea of how you were sitting matches the reality.
3. Again without using the mirror try and sit as symmetrically as possible.
4. Using the mirror once again check to see whether:
   (a) your head is on one side;
   (b) one shoulder is higher than the other;
   (c) you are not leaning over to one side;
   (d) your legs and feet are also symmetrical.

Repeat this every day for a week or two, writing down any observations, and you will soon see your pattern of 'use' emerging. It is a good idea always to remember that human beings were not designed to sit for long periods of time, and very few chair designers really understand the mechanics of the human body. Therefore if you do have to sit for hours on end make sure you get up and walk around every so often. There may be times when you could walk to nearby places instead of using the car.

It is worth noting that the spine is under much more stress when sitting than when standing. Most chairs, especially car seats, slope backwards encouraging the sitter to slump forward, and you have to hold yourself up to counteract this effect. You can, however, buy chairs that have an adjustable seat so that you can actually have it sloping *forwards*. This helps to prevent the slumping or the sinking down into the hips that so often occurs. You can produce the same effect by placing a two inch piece of wood or a couple of telephone books under the back legs of any kitchen chair. Try it for yourself.

A whole range of seat accessories has been designed and developed by engineer and chiropractor John Gorman, whose address can be found at the back of this book.

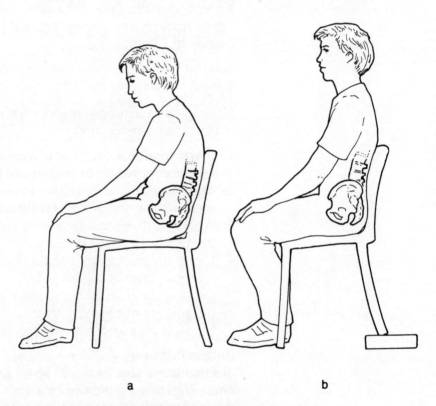

a   b

Fig. 10a   A common sitting position (slumped).

Fig. 10b   An improved sitting position (sloping forward).

Chapter 7

THE MECHANICS OF MOVEMENT

It is essential that the peoples of civilization should comprehend the value of their inheritance, that outcome of the long process of evolution which will enable them to govern the uses of their own physical mechanisms. By and through consciousness and the application of a reasoning intelligence, man may rise above the powers of all disease and physical disabilities. This triumph is not to be won in sleep, in trance, in submission, in paralysis, or in anaesthesia, but in a clear, open-eyed, reasoning, deliberate consciousness by mankind, the transcendent inheritance of a conscious mind.

FREDERICK MATTHIAS ALEXANDER

Have you ever stopped for a moment to think about how you actually move around this world? And is it the easiest and most efficient way of going about your activities? Most people do not give the subject any thought whatsoever; in fact it is so alien that at first it is difficult to comprehend what is being asked of us.

In reality we consist of 206 bones placed one on top of the other. These are suspended by a 'suit' of muscles which holds us together and, by maintaining a certain tone, keeps us in an upright position. At the very top of this structure is the head which weighs approximately 15 pounds (7 kilogrammes).

Exercise

Gather together objects weighing 15 pounds; for instance seven bags of sugar or three bags of potatoes. Place them in a container (a box or a bag) and you have the equivalent weight of your own head. It is a very surprising experience, when you realize that you are balancing this weight every moment of your waking life.

That is not all. The head is actually set off-balance on top of our spines; therefore if we relax the neck muscles the head always drops forward. If you watch someone falling asleep sitting in a chair the head invariably drops forward on to the chest. So not only are we trying to balance a 15-pound head, but also coping with the fact that its point of balance is not under its centre of gravity (*see* Fig. 11).

Fig. 11 Diagram of the skull and the top vertebrae showing the pivot point and the centre of gravity of the head.

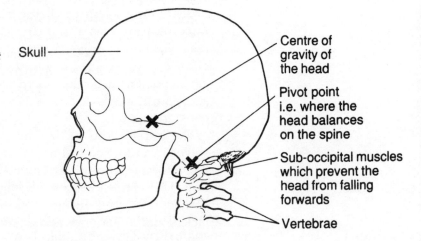

Skull

Centre of gravity of the head

Pivot point i.e. where the head balances on the spine

Sub-occipital muscles which prevent the head from falling forwards

Vertebrae

Exercise

Take a dinner plate – one you wouldn't mind breaking! Place your finger in the middle of the plate (its centre of gravity), and try to balance the plate using just that one finger.

Now repeat the process but this time place your finger two inches away from the centre. This is exactly the same relationship as the head to the neck.

At first this does not seem to make any sense. Surely if we are to carry around such an incredible weight on top of our spines then it would be sensible for nature to have placed our heads in balance. It is an intriguing puzzle. The answer is simple, and yet at the same time brilliant.

Exercise

Spend a moment seeing whether you can solve the mystery of why the head is always off-balance in this way.

IMBALANCE OF THE HEAD

The reason that the pivot point of the head is behind its centre of gravity is that, in order to move, all a person has to do is relax the sub-occipital muscles (at the back of the head). The head will then go forward slightly and because of its weight will take the whole body into movement. In other words, in order to move, a human being has only to let go of the tension in certain muscles and a complex reflex system will do the rest. Most other movements require effort, and the maximum effort is needed at the beginning of the action. For example, a car needs most power when it starts off from a stationary position; it needs relatively little energy to keep it going at a constant speed.

The implications of this are profound. If we can use ourselves in a more co-ordinated way, our movements will need less effort and thus give us much more energy at the end of the day. This can lead to a more harmonious way of life as most conflicts and stressful situations are triggered off by fatigue or lack of vitality. Friends and relatives of Alexander pupils often report a marked change of temperament after only a few lessons. I have heard many comments like, 'John is much more easy-going than he used to be and in fact is a much nicer man to live with.'

So the principle of the Alexander Technique is to use our bodies as nature intended; that is, to *decrease* muscular tension in order to move, and not (as most of us do) to increase tension in our muscles. This concept of having to make an effort for movement is reinforced throughout our lives by parents and teachers who tell us: 'You won't get anywhere in this world without making a great deal of effort.' Because of this we subconsciously make life much harder than it really needs to be, which is apparent both physically and mentally. By 'letting go' into movement, it is possible to experience how easy and effortless many things can be. Once this starts to permeate our subconscious mind, we are able to be more relaxed in everything we do.

THE INSTABILITY OF THE HUMAN FRAME

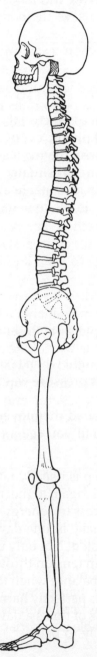

As I have said, the skeleton, which consists of over two hundred bones assembled one on top of the other, is inherently unstable. It is similar to a pile of children's building blocks – the higher the blocks are placed, the more unstable they become until they actually fall over. This, together with the fact that the head is off-balance, indicates that we have to do very little in order to move. We are designed to 'fall' into movement and when infants first begin to learn to walk they do just that. They constantly look as though they are about to fall flat on their faces, yet they save themselves just in time by the reflex action of their legs.

Throughout the years, however, because of our unconscious fear of falling we tend to stabilize ourselves by tensing up our muscular system. This of course affects our whole physiological system, rendering our reflexes relatively ineffective. As a result we use excessive muscular effort to perform the same action that ought to be done by our reflexes alone.

> Each faculty acquires fitness for its function by performing its function; and if its function is performed for it by a substituted agency, none of the required adjustments of nature takes place, but the nature becomes deformed to fit the artificial arrangements instead of the natural arrangements.
>
> Herbert Spencer

In short, if we do not use ourselves in the way that nature intended we start to use our muscular mechanisms in a way that will invariably cause unnecessary rigidity of some parts of the body, and an over-relaxation of others. This undue rigidity is always found in those parts of the muscular system which are forced to perform duties other than those intended by nature, and are therefore ill-adapted for their function.

Fig. 12   We are in fact 206 bones placed one on top of the other.

WALKING

When we bear in mind the principles described earlier, walking becomes an action whereby we work *with* gravity rather than against it. Walking is a process of letting go of certain muscles that connect the head to the rest of the body, thus allowing the head to move very slightly forward. Since the rest of the body is already in a state of instability, it will then move by falling forward. As soon as the body detects even the smallest amount of movement the reflex mechanism will automatically send a leg out in front to save the body from falling over.

An important principle emerges when examining the natural way of walking, namely that:

THE HEAD ALWAYS LEADS ANY MOVEMENT

It is essential to understand this in order to practise the Technique. Whether it be a snake or an elephant, every animal moves with its head leading; which is why the main sensory organs (eyes, ears, nose and tongue) are all situated in the head. At first this may seem like an obvious statement, but few human beings apply this principle in movement.

Exercise

1. Stand in front of a mirror.
2. Take a step forward.
3. Ask yourself: 'What did I have to do when taking that step?'
4. Notice if you moved to the left or the right when taking the step. (If you did it is likely that excess pressure was placed on the hip.)
5. Ask yourself: 'What part of me initiated the movement?'
6. Repeat the exercise several times until you see a pattern emerging.

As you have probably discovered, a step is usually taken by lifting the leg with the thigh muscles against the pull of gravity. This of course expends unnecessary energy and if you think about how many steps you take in one day alone you will realize how much energy is wasted. Not only is there a waste of energy, but also an increase in tension throughout the whole structure simply to maintain balance when the foot is raised from the ground. This tension is perfectly harmless if occasional, but when it occurs hundreds of times a day it will inevitably lead to rigidity and eventually to pain.

Fig. 13 Ungainly ways of walking.

Fig. 13a Moving in disconnected sections.

Fig. 13b Walking with hips forward and head dropped.

The arrows indicate the direction of movement of parts of the body

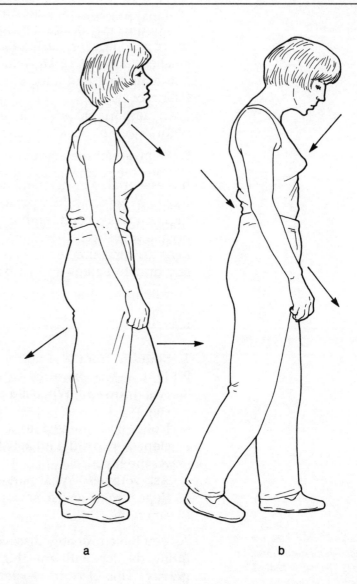

a   b

Exercise

1. Allow yourself to fall forward and save yourself by taking a step.
2. Notice if you have a preference as to which leg you use to save yourself.
3. Are you still inclined to lift the leg rather than let it work by reflex?
4. As you begin to walk, try to notice if you are walking on the outside or the inside of the foot. (There should be fairly

equal pressure on both sides of the foot, and if anything a slight inclination towards the outside; because excess pressure on the inside of the foot will invariably lead to the collapse of the arch.) NB Any changes that might come about must be done by applying your direction (see chapter 10.)

5. Be aware as you walk whether your feet have a tendency to point in or out. (It is possible and indeed highly likely that one foot may differ from the other.)
6. Be aware of the amount of pressure that is present when your foot comes into contact with the ground.

I cannot stress too much the importance of not *trying* to change anything; this will always result in an increase of muscular tension and make the situation worse. A change will take place simply by making your habit conscious. This change may not be immediately apparent; you may not notice the difference for a few days or even weeks, so try to be patient.

BENDING DOWN

When bending down to pick objects up many people only bend at the hip joint (that is where the femur connects into the pelvis). (*See* Figure 14a.) This puts an enormous strain on the back muscles especially those in the lower back area. Without realizing it, they are actually picking up half their body weight in addition to the weight of the object. For example, if a person weighing 12 stone (76 kilogrammes) picks up an object which weighs 2 stone (12.7 kilogrammes) without bending their

Fig. 14a   This is how the majority of people bend over to pick up things. The whole body is under stress because the top of the body is no longer over its support (the feet).

Fig. 14b   Picking up an object – the position of mechanical advantage. As the person lowers herself she is in balance and therefore not putting an excessive strain on her structure. This position is often seen in children but hardly ever in adults.

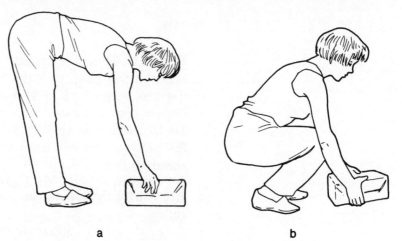

a   b

knees, they are in fact lifting an extra 7 stone (44.35 kilogrammes) in body weight with their lower back muscles, which will of course cause considerable tension. This sort of misuse nearly always leads to lower back pain, or in extreme cases to a 'slipped disc'. If you ever watch professional weight-lifters on television, you will see that they always squat when bending (as young children do) using mainly their very powerful thigh and buttock muscles, and not the muscles of the back.

As you can see from Figure 14b this person is perfectly poised and nicely balanced as she lowers herself. Alexander called this the 'position of mechanical advantage'.

THE POSITION OF MECHANICAL ADVANTAGE

The 'position of mechanical advantage' is a position devised by Alexander to keep the body in a state of equilibrium and ease while performing an action that requires a lowering of stature. He describes the position thus in his first book *Man's Supreme Inheritance*:

> By my system of obtaining the position of 'mechanical advantage', a perfect system of natural internal massage is rendered possible, such as never before has been attained by orthodox methods, a system which is extraordinarily beneficial in breaking up toxic accumulation; thus avoiding evils which arise from auto-intoxication.

Exercise

1. Place a book on the ground in front of you.
2. Without thinking, pick the book up in your natural way (i.e. the way which feels most comfortable to you).
3. Repeat several times.
4. Try to notice how you bend down. Do you only bend from the pelvis or do you use your ankle, knee and hip joints simultaneously?
5. Try squatting. If you find this hard just see how far down you can go. Do not force yourself to do more than you can manage. You may need to steady yourself at first by holding on to a nearby chair or table.

As you become more aware of yourself in different situations, like taking the milk from the fridge or picking up the post in the morning, you will begin to notice a change in the way that you move. Everyday activities become much easier, which of course will reflect in your attitude to life in general.

At first this new way of moving may feel strange or even abnormal, because it is outside your habit patterns. However, within a short space of time the new way becomes natural and the old habits begin to feel uncoordinated and clumsy.

FROM STANDING TO SITTING

A common habit is to fall backwards when sitting down. This excites our fear reflexes unduly and causes us to tense unnecessarily. Also the legs do not get the exercise they need to keep them in a fit condition. A better way to sit down is to go into a bend as in Figure 15 and then gently allow your sitting bones to reach the chair. You should always be able to change your mind and get up at a moment's notice. If you have difficulty with this, simply sit down in the chair as though it was not there and in this way you will always be in balance.

Also when standing up we can put enormous strain on our entire structure (*see* Figure 16).

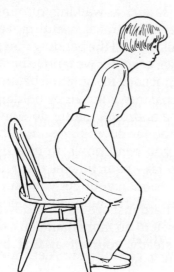

Fig. 15 In order to sit in a co-ordinated way the head needs to be over the feet until the person reaches the chair.

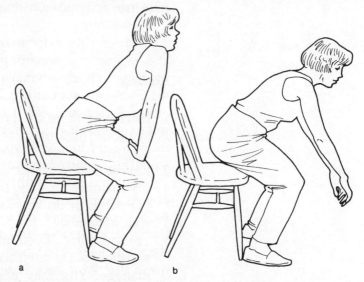

a   b

Fig. 16 When standing up we can put enormous strain upon our entire structure. Beware of pushing (figure 16a) or of swinging up (figure 16b).

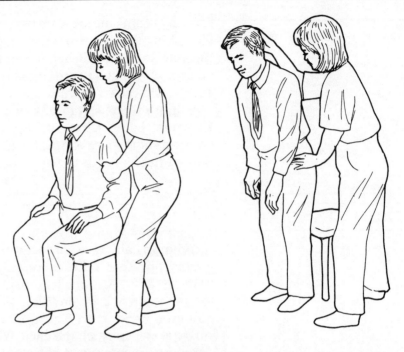

Fig. 17   An Alexander Teacher helps the pupil to move in new ways, putting less strain on the body. The teacher encourages the pupil to go 'up' when sitting, and to keep length while bending.

Exercise

Apart from natural forms of exercise such as walking, running and swimming, squatting is one of the most useful movements your body can make. As children, all the bending down we do involves squatting, but as we get older we tend to bend our knees less and less. If you are not used to squatting be sure not to overdo it. You can help to balance yourself by holding on to a firm fixture in your home and then gently do some squatting, taking care not to go too far down to begin with.

You could also try this when you bend down to pick up objects from the floor. Be sure to take your time as this will help you to observe any excess tension in your body. Be sure that your ankle, knee and hip joints bend simultaneously, and that you keep your back straight, although this does not mean that your back is always vertical.

If you have any problems be sure to consult your Alexander teacher.

Chapter 8

Faulty Sensory Perception

The fault, dear Brutus, is not in our stars,
But in ourselves.

WILLIAM SHAKESPEARE *Julius Caesar*

The main difficulty people have when starting to practise the Alexander Technique is the very difficulty experienced by Alexander himself, namely that they are suffering from an unreliable sensory appreciation of themselves. This simply means that their proprioception (the sense that tells us where parts of our body are in relation to other parts and in space) has become faulty and is actually giving false information.

> There must be, in the first place, a clear realization by the pupil that he suffers from a defect or defects needing eradication. In the second place, the teacher must make a lucid diagnosis of such defects and decide upon the means of dealing with them. He (the pupil) acknowledges that he suffers from mental delusions regarding his physical acts and that his sensory appreciation, or kinaesthesis, is defective and misleading. In other words, he realizes that his sense register of the amount of muscular tension needed to accomplish even a simple act of everyday life is faulty and harmful, and his mental conception of such conditions as relaxation and concentration is impossible in practical application.
>
> For there can be no doubt that man on the subconscious plane now relies too much on a debauched sense of feeling or of sense-appreciation for the guidance of his psychophysical mechanism, and that he is gradually becoming more and more overbalanced emotionally, with very harmful and far reaching results.
>
> Frederick Matthias Alexander

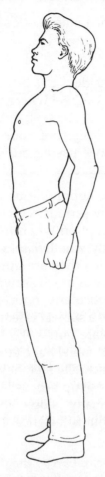

In short, what we are actually doing and what we think we are doing may be two totally different things.

Exercise

To demonstrate the above:
1. Without looking at your feet, place them nine inches apart pointing them straight ahead so that they are parallel to each other.
2. Now look at your feet to see if the intended position of your feet matches the real position.
3. This time look at your feet and place them nine inches apart so that they are parallel.
4. What do they feel like?

Try this exercise on as many people as possible noticing that the position of the feet can vary enormously from person to person. Try another exercise:

1. Ask a friend to sit on a chair.
2. Place your hand on the lumbar arch of the spine.
3. Ask your friend to sit up straight.
4. Observe how they arch their back by shortening the spine therefore becoming bowed in shape instead of straight.

Fig. 18 Faulty sensory perception. The man thinks he is standing up straight when in fact he is leaning backwards with his back in the shape of a bow.

THE KINAESTHETIC SENSE

This is a term mentioned time and time again in connection with the Alexander Technique. The kinaesthetic sense sends messages to the brain whenever there is movement of the joints and muscles. These sensations send impulses along nerves to the brain, and thus inform it of the location of the limb in space and of the relative position to each other of individual muscles and muscle-groups, and of the joints.

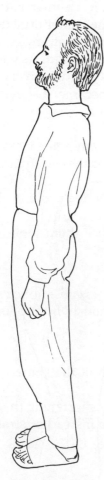

Fig. 19 The man thinks he is upright but is leaning back.

Exercise

To understand in a practical way what the kinaesthetic sense is:

1. Close your eyes.
2. Slowly raise your left arm out to the side.
3. Without opening your eyes see if you can feel where your arm is in space.
4. If you have been able to locate the position of your arm without looking then you must have used your kinaesthetic sense to do so.

If, as Alexander discovered, this sense is supplying us with false information then the implications are serious. The most common example of faulty sensory perception when teaching, is the pupil's inability to tell correctly whether they are upright when standing. Many people think they are upright when in fact they are leaning backwards by as much as twenty degrees. In group situations this is particularly noticeable because everyone else can see clearly that a subject is leaning backwards, yet they are convinced they are not.

This belief system is so entrenched that when I have guided the person into an upright position they actually feel they are leaning forward, so much so that they tense up because they think they are about to fall over. Since many people spend most of their waking hours completely out of balance, their muscles are constantly under strain.

RIGHTS AND WRONGS

In order to make the necessary changes in ourselves, to bring about a new and improved way of moving, we need to do the very thing that feels wrong. Alexander once said:

> The right thing to do would be the last thing we should do, left to ourselves, because it would be the last thing we should think it would be the right thing to do. Everyone wants to be right, but no one stops to consider if their idea of right is right. When people are wrong, the thing that is right is bound to be wrong to them.

So the problem is, in fact, quite complex. It is human nature to move, sit or stand in a way that feels most comfortable. We would not dream of moving in a way that feels strange or even alien to us, and yet this is exactly what is required. As you will remember, Alexander stumbled across this discovery only because he was using a mirror. He became disheartened

Fig. 20   An Alexander Teacher will gently alter the pupil's muscle tone in order to release tension.

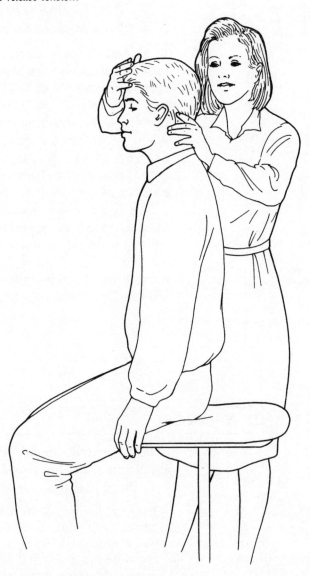

when he realized he was doing exactly the opposite of what he had intended to do; that he was trying to put his head forward and up, when in reality he was pulling his head back and down in an even more pronounced way than before.

Alexander used to advise his pupils to 'try and feel wrong', because in that way the pupil would have a chance of doing the right action. For this reason it is highly recommended initially to take a course of lessons because it is so easy to increase muscular tension and aggravate any problem (or potential problem) that you have. Because he has been highly trained and is also an objective observer, the teacher can easily detect any extra tension that may occur when you are trying to put something right. He can also impart an experience of lightness and ease of movement which can be used as a point of reference when experimenting with your own movements.

We are conditioned from an early age to be right. We get rewards when we are right and punishments when we are wrong and, like Pavlov's dogs, we begin to form fixed ideas about what is right and wrong and what is good and bad. As we grow up we form ideas based on what is taught to us at school and by our parents, and are often discouraged from thinking for ourselves. Look at history! There was a time when the people of Europe 'knew' that the world was flat. They were so convinced of this that anyone who said otherwise and threatened their belief system was ridiculed and often called insane. It was not until Christopher Columbus had sailed right around the world that people would admit they were wrong. In the same way, we walk around with many incorrect concepts about ourselves and would challenge anyone to tell us otherwise!

It is important to have an open mind and a good sense of humour when trying to find your way through this maze of illusions and realities. A pupil will often come to a point of confusion when he begins to realize that ideas which he had thought to be true were actually based on a false premise. However, this confusion is soon replaced by realization after realization of what is true and what is not. This is summed up in a line from *Illusions* by Richard Bach:

> There is no such thing as a problem without a gift for you in its hands.

To give some further examples of faulty sensory feelings try the following exercises:

Exercise 1

1. Close your eyes.
2. Raise the index finger of your right hand so that it is at eye level and in line with your right ear.
3. Raise the index finger of your left hand so that it is at eye level and in line with your left ear.
4. Keeping your eyes closed, try to line up your fingers so that the two are level and are pointing straight up into the air.
5. Open your eyes and see how close the reality is to the feeling.

Exercise 2

1. Ask a friend to stand in front of you with their eyes shut.
2. Ask them to raise their arms so that they are level with the shoulders.
3. Check to see (a) if one arm is higher than the other; and (b) if both arms are in fact level with the shoulders.

Exercise 3

1. Close your eyes.
2. Clap your hands so that your hands meet in an even and symmetrical way (i.e. the thumbs and fingers are all touching their counterparts so that their tops are at the same height).
3. Open your eyes to see how close you are.

The implications, and indeed the effects, of faulty sensory perception on the human structure can be seen very clearly in old age, when many people have become bent or twisted as their body tries to cope with their lack of co-ordination. The only way a pupil can achieve any progress toward making their unreliable sensory feelings more reliable is to accept that during a course of Alexander lessons they may well experience ways of moving that initially feel very unnatural to them. In a comparatively short period of time, however, the new way of being will begin to feel normal and old habits will start to feel clumsy by comparison.

It is important to point out that the phrase 'unreliable feelings' refers only to sensory feelings and not to emotional feelings. It can be said, however, that the faulty perception of ourselves is bound to affect our physical state, which will in turn influence our day-to-day emotional condition. Our reason then becomes completely dominated by our emotions to the point where our perception of what is true becomes distorted, thus influencing our ability to discriminate between right and wrong. In this way a vicious cycle is set up.

Exercise

Stand side on to a mirror and in what you think is an upright posture. Make sure that you are standing as straight as you possibly can. Then check by using the mirror to see whether your feelings of being straight match the reality. If they do not, stand in a posture that you can see is straight and ask yourself whether you are perceiving yourself in a reliable way. Be sure to take time over this exercise to observe as much detail as possible. To make this exercise easier you may like to use 2 mirrors at an angle to one another.

Chapter 9

INHIBITION

We are nature's unique experiment to make the rational intelligence prove sounder than the reflex.
Success or failure of this experiment depends on the basic human ability to impose a delay between the stimulus and the response.
BRONOWSKI

The word 'inhibition' has been commonly used to describe a self-imposed suppression of behaviour or emotions ever since Sigmund Freud used the term in this way in his writings on psychoanalysis.

The actual dictionary definition of 'inhibition' is:

'THE RESTRAINT OF DIRECT EXPRESSION
OF AN INSTINCT.'

Alexander realized that in order to bring about a desirable change in the use of his body he would first have to inhibit (or stop) his habitual, instinctive responses to a given stimulus. *By stopping for a moment before an action takes place we have time to use our reasoning powers to check which is the most efficient and appropriate way of performing such an action.* This is a vital step towards having the power to choose freely on every level.

Before the brain can be used as an instrument for **action**, it has to be used as an instrument for **inaction**. The ability to **delay** (**pause**) our responses until we are adequately prepared is what is meant by **inhibition**.

This moment of pausing before acting has nothing to do with **freezing** or **suppression**, neither is it about performing actions slowly.

INSTINCTIVE INHIBITION

The best example of natural and instinctive inhibition is the cat. You can observe this even in a domestic cat, when it first sees a mouse. It does not immediately rush and capture its prey, but waits until the appropriate moment in order to achieve the highest chance of success.

> A cat inhibits the desire to spring prematurely, and controls to a deliberate end its eagerness for the instant gratification of a natural appetite.
>
> Frederick Matthias Alexander

It is an interesting fact that while cats are fine examples of inhibition and control, they are at the same time one of the fastest creatures on earth. The cat's ability to pause is instinctual; in other words, it is an automatic function of the subconscious brain. Man, by contrast, has this potential subject to conscious control, and it is this difference which defines a clear line between man and the animal world.

Alexander firmly believed that we have to delay our instantaneous response to the many stimuli that bombard us each day, if we are to cope with our rapidly changing environment. As our direct dependence on the body for subsistence has decreased, our instinct has become increasingly unreliable so that it is now necessary, through the use of inhibition, to employ our conscious powers to fill the gap.

CONSCIOUS INHIBITION

If we are ever to change our habitual responses to given stimuli we have to make a conscious decision to refuse to act in our old automatic and unconscious patterns; that is, to say 'no' to our ingrained habits of use.

By inhibiting our initial instinctive action we have the choice to make an entirely different decision. Inhibition is an essential and integral step when practising the Technique, and Alexander summarized it thus:

> Boiled down it all comes to inhibiting a particular reaction to a given stimulus – but no one will see it that way. They will see it as getting in and out of a chair the right way. It is nothing of the kind. It is that a pupil decides what he will, or will not, consent to do.

There are many old sayings and proverbs that point to the wisdom of thought before action:

- Look before you leap.
- Think on the end before you begin.
- Second thoughts are best.
- More haste, less speed.
- Good and quickly seldom meet.
- Think first, then speak.
- Be led by reason (Greek proverb).
- Life is *not* an emergency.

If you are able to prevent yourself from performing your habitual actions then you are half-way to your goal. To refrain from an action is as much an act as actually performing an activity, because in both cases the nervous system is employed. It is also possible, and indeed desirable, to inhibit any unwanted habits and tendencies, not only before an action takes place, but also during any given activity.

Exercises

1. Every time the telephone or the doorbell rings, pause just for two seconds before answering. (You may find this simple exercise harder to do than it first seems.)
2. Whenever you find yourself in a heated discussion or an argument, try counting backwards from ten to one before responding. (As well as being a useful exercise in inhibition it will give you time to think about what you really want to convey.)
3. Choose a simple activity, such as cleaning your teeth or doing the washing-up, and occasionally stop completely for a moment or two and be aware of any excess tension you may be holding in your body. If you do this each day for several days running you are likely to find that the areas of tension will be the same each day. Try, if possible, to let go of any tension that you feel and then proceed with the activity, noticing whether you feel any different as a result.
4. (a) Place a chair in front of a mirror.
   (b) Stand up and sit down in your normal way and see if you can notice any habitual tendencies (i.e. any one thing that occurs every time), but do not worry if you can't.
   (c) Repeat the above, but this time pause for a moment or

two before carrying out the action, while you consciously refuse to sit down or stand up in your normal way. Soon you will see that there are many different ways of performing the same action.

(d) See whether you notice any differences between the first and second way of performing the action. (You may see a difference in the mirror or you may feel a difference on a sensory level.)

You may need to carry out the above exercises a few times before you are aware of the differences.

One of the most noticeable tendencies that Alexander observed in himself was that he constantly tightened his neck muscles, in particular the sterno-cleido-mastoid, and the trapezius. Initially he presumed that this phenomenon was merely a personal idiosyncrasy, but later observations showed him that this was not the case at all – this tensing-up of the neck muscles was practically universal.

This habit invariably leads to a pulling back of the head on to the spine thus compressing the intervertebral discs and shortening the structure. This constant pressure on the spine is one of the main reasons why most people 'shrink' with age. The pulling back of the head also interferes dramatically with what Alexander called the 'Primary Control'. As mentioned in Chapter 2 this is simply a term for a system of reflexes which takes place in the neck area and has the power to control all the other reflexes to direct the body in a co-ordinated and balanced way. It is called 'primary' because if this reflex action is interfered with all the other reflexes throughout the body will be affected.

If we are truly pulling our heads back habitually and interfering with the Primary Control, then the implications are serious indeed. Our co-ordination and balance will be severely affected, and we will be forced to hold ourselves in a rigid fashion to stop ourselves from falling over. In other words, when we come to move we will actually be working against ourselves.

A learner driver who grips the steering wheel too tightly with one hand may have difficulty moving the wheel with the other. As a driving instructor I encountered many people who thought there was something wrong with the car because the wheel would not move very easily!

EXPERIMENTAL EVIDENCE

In the mid–1920s, Rudolph Magnus, a professor of pharmacology at the University of Utrecht, became interested in exploring the role our physiological mechanisms play in affecting our mental and emotional well-being. Magnus was struck by the central function of the reflexes that governed the position of an animal's head in relation to the rest of its body and to its environment. With his colleagues, he performed a series of experiments to establish the nature and function of postural reflexes throughout the body. He wrote over three hundred papers on the subject, pointing to the fact that it was the head–neck reflexes that were the central controlling mechanism responsible for orienting the animal to his environment, both in assuming a posture for a particular purpose and also in restoring the animal to a resting posture after an action.

Magnus's experiments confirmed what Alexander had discovered in himself a quarter of a century earlier: that in all animals the mechanism of the body is set up in such a way that the head leads a movement and then the body follows. In retrospect this seems to be an obvious statement because all the senses are in the head and if we follow our senses as we are designed to do then our head will automatically lead the way. This phenomenon occurs naturally in all animals with the exception of man, in whom it can clearly be seen that the head is constantly being thrown back when a movement takes place.

Exercise

To demonstrate that the head is pulled back by excess tension of the neck muscles during a movement, follow these steps:

1. Sit in a chair.
2. Place your left hand on the left side of the neck, and the right hand on the right side of the neck, so that the two middle fingers are just touching at the back of the neck (at the base of the skull).
3. Stand up.
4. Then sit down again.
5. By being aware of your hands at the time of sitting and standing you will be able to detect any pulling back of the

head. Watch for a feeling that the neck is being pressed into the hands. This indicates neck tension and the head being pulled back.

6. Perform the exercise several times as you may well notice more tension on the second or third repetition.

The other major discovery made by Magnus was what he called 'the righting reflex'. He noticed that after an action which requires extra tension has taken place (for example, a cat leaping onto a table) a set of 'righting reflexes' come into play which restore the animal (or human) to its normal composed posture. The relationship of the head, neck and back is an essential factor when this righting mechanism is in operation. Therefore it is true to say that when a person stiffens their neck muscles and pulls their head back, not only are they obstructing the body's natural co-ordination, but the body is also prevented from returning to its natural state of ease and equilibrium.

> What a piece of work is a man! how noble in reason! how infinite in faculty! in form and moving how express and admirable! in action how like an angel! in apprehension how like a god! the beauty of the world! the paragon of animals!
>
> William Shakespeare (*Hamlet*)

Alexander once commented on the above passage, saying:

> These words seem to me now to be contradicted by what I have discovered in myself and others. For what could be less 'noble in reason', less 'infinite in faculty' than that man, despite his potentialities, should have fallen into such error in the use of himself, and in this way brought about such a lowering in his standard of functioning that in everything he attempts to accomplish, these harmful conditions tend to become more and more exaggerated? In consequence, how many people are there today of whom it may be said, as regards their use of themselves, 'in form and moving how express and admirable'? Can we any longer consider man in this regard 'The paragon of animals'?

Yet if we are able to inhibit this unconscious habit of tensing up our neck muscles, then this will free our whole body to perform actions in such a way that they become as much a joy to watch as they are to carry out.

Exercise

Another exercise to try is to stand up with both arms resting by your sides. Take a moment to be aware of what they feel like. Do they feel the same or does one arm feel longer, heavier, freer, than the other?

Without thinking raise one arm up to the side so that it is level with your shoulder. Hold it there for a moment or two and then relax the arm back down to the side. Do exactly the same with the other arm, but first inhibit your action so that you can be aware in more detail of raising the second arm up.

Notice if you can feel any difference in your two arms after you have performed this exercise. Often people experience a feeling of lightness in the second arm that is not present in the first. Repeat the same exercise, but using opposite arms.

Chapter 10

DIRECTION

You come to learn to inhibit and to direct your activity. You learn, first, to inhibit the habitual reaction to certain classes of stimuli, and second, to direct yourself consciously in such a way as to affect certain muscular pulls, which processes bring about a new reaction to these stimuli.

FREDERICK MATTHIAS ALEXANDER

During Alexander's years of experimentation he was led to a long consideration of the whole question of directing his body. He had to admit that he had never once given any thought to how he directed himself in activity. He had used himself habitually in the way that felt 'natural' and 'right' to him. So at this point he started to formulate actual instructions or orders to give himself to make up for this lack of natural direction.

To give directions is:

A PROCESS WHICH INVOLVES PROJECTING MESSAGES FROM THE BRAIN TO THE BODY'S MECHANISMS AND CONDUCTING THE ENERGY NECESSARY FOR THE USE OF THESE MECHANISMS.

It is possible to direct *specific* parts of yourself (for example, you can think of your fingers lengthening); or to direct your *whole* self (such as when thinking of your entire structure lengthening). You can also direct yourself through space by consciously deciding where you are going and how you intend to get there.

THE MAIN DIRECTIONS

Alexander realized that the root cause of many problems was that the over-tightening of the neck muscles caused an interference with the 'Primary Control', which in turn threw the whole body out of balance. He realized that the first and most important step was to give the necessary directions to ensure a lessening of tension in the neck area so that the normal functioning of the 'Primary Control' would be restored.

The directions he devised were:

1. Allow the neck to be free

so that

2. The head can go forward and upward

in order that

3. The back can lengthen and widen.

As there are many Alexander teachers today these orders may vary a little. For example:

1. *Allow your neck to be free* is sometimes changed to:
   Let the neck be free, *or*
   Think of the neck as being free, *or*
   Think of the neck muscles releasing.
   Think of not stiffening the neck, *or*
   Relax the neck (Alexander himself initially used this order but he changed the wording when he found that his pupils tended to over-relax their neck muscles.)

2. *The head can go forward and upwards* is often changed to:
   Think of allowing the head going forward and up, *or*
   Let the head go forward and up, *or*
   Allow the head to go forwards and upwards, *or*
   Think of not pulling the head backwards and downwards.

3. *The back can lengthen and widen* can also become:
   Think of the back lengthening and widening, *or*
   Allow the back to lengthen and widen, *or*
   Think of not shortening and narrowing the back, *or*
   Let the torso lengthen and widen.

Allow the neck to be free

The purpose of this instruction is to eliminate the excess tension that is almost always present in the muscles of the neck. This is essential if the head is to be free in relation to the rest of the body, in order for the 'Primary Control' to perform its natural function. This should always be the first direction given, because unless the 'Primary Control' is able to organize the rest of the body, any other directions will be relatively ineffective.

Allow the head to go forward and upward

This direction helps the mechanisms of the body to function naturally and freely. As we saw in Chapter 7 (The Mechanics of Movement), the head is balanced in such a way that when the neck muscles are released the head goes slightly forward which takes the whole body into movement. If you think only of the head going forward and not upward, it would invariably drop downward causing increased muscular tension in the neck area. It is important to realize that the forward direction is the head going forward *on the spine* (as if you are about to nod your head affirmatively). The upward direction of the head is *away from the spine* and not away from the earth, although these may well be the same when the structure is upright (*see* Figure 21).

Fig. 21 Diagram of the head showing the directions of head movement.

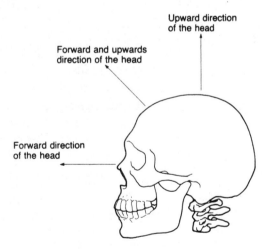

Upward direction
of the head

Forward and upwards
direction of the head

Forward direction
of the head

Allow the back to lengthen and widen

Since it is the spine that shortens because of excess muscular tension when the head is pulled back, this direction will encourage a lengthening of the whole structure. In fact, many people who practise the Alexander Technique actually increase in height by an inch or more! The reason a widening direction is included is that it is easy for a narrowing to occur while the lengthening process is taking place.

These three primary directions are in themselves very simple and straightforward. However, because of our 'debauched kinaesthesia' (a favourite term of Alexander's which can be used to impress people at parties!), they can be confusing when first practised. This is partly because they are so simple and we are used to thinking in a more complicated way; it is hard to believe that the solution to what may have been a longstanding problem can indeed be so simple. We live in a fast-moving world, and when results do not happen immediately we presume that we are doing something wrong. Be patient and observant, and realize that you are changing the habits of a lifetime.

It is strongly advised that when you start giving directions you have at least a few lessons from a trained Alexander teacher to make sure you are on the right track.

SECONDARY DIRECTIONS

There are many secondary directions, too numerous to mention. Whereas the main or primary directions can be applied universally, the secondary directions may be applied to certain conditions or ailments. For example, if a person comes to me suffering from rounded shoulders I may give them an instruction to: 'Think of your shoulders going away from each other'; or if someone comes to me with arthritic fingers, I may ask them to: 'Think of your fingers lengthening'.

Here are some examples of secondary directions commonly used in the teaching of the Technique:

When sitting

Think of the shoulders going away from each other.
Think of the sitting bones releasing into the chair.
Think of the feet lengthening and widening.
Think of a lengthening from the wrist to the elbow.
Think of the shoulders dropping.

Think of the elbows dropping.
Think of the weight of the legs dropping through the feet.
Think of the hands lengthening and widening.
Think of the fingers lengthening.
Think of the toes lengthening.
Think about not arching the back.
Think of the rib-cage dropping.

When standing

Most of the directions above, plus:

Think of a lengthening between the feet and the head.
Think of letting your weight go evenly through the soles of
   your feet.
Think of not bracing the knees back.
Think of not pushing the hips forward.
Think of lengthening between the navel and the upper part of
   the chest.
Think of letting go of tension in the buttocks.
Think of the arms dropping from the shoulders.
Think of a connection between the head and the feet.

When walking

Again many of the directions above, plus:

Think of the knees going away from each other.
Think of the knees going over the toes.
Think of the release of the left shoulder from the right hip.
Think of the release of the right shoulder from the left hip.
Think of the weight being transferred from the heel to the
   toes.
Think of the torso coming up out of the hips.

There are many more to suit an individual's needs, but the
primary directions *always* precede any secondary direction
that may be given.

The words 'think of' may often be substituted by the word
'allow' or 'think of allowing' depending on the teacher's or
pupil's preference. It is interesting to see if they have different
effects on the body. The most important thing to remember at

all times is to bring about a change by thinking alone, and not to try and *do* anything to bring about a change. As I have said repeatedly, when you try to *do* anything it always increases the muscular tension, which is the very opposite of what you are trying to achieve.

The last type of direction is thinking of directing your body as a whole entity: 'In what direction am I going in?'

Exercise

1. Look at an object of your choice.
2. Without taking your eyes off it think of your eyes getting closer and closer to the object.
3. As the head begins to move towards the object let the rest of the body follow. This will show you how the head can lead the body.

> There is no such thing as a right position, but there is such a thing as a right direction.
>
> Frederick Matthias Alexander

People often associate the Alexander Technique with putting parts of the body in certain positions, but it is exactly the opposite of this; it is that the head retains a freedom from the rest of the body no matter what position it is in.

THOUGHT AFFECTS FUNCTIONING

It is very hard for us to believe that thinking alone can bring about such radical changes in a person, but as a teacher of the Technique I have witnessed this change in hundreds of people. It really does work. You can demonstrate the effect thought has on your organism by performing the following exercises:

Exercise 1

Try this one on yourself and then on a friend.

1. The actual weight of an arm is approximately eight pounds, that is about four bags of sugar. So with this thought in mind begin to raise your arms up slowly to the sides.

2. It should take you about half a minute to raise your arms up until they are horizontal. Keep thinking of the actual weight of your arms the whole time.
3. Hold your arms at the horizontal position for another half a minute or so to get a sense of how heavy they really are (four bags of sugar in each arm).
4. Slowly lower your arms back down to your sides.
5. Take a minute or two and make a note (either mental or on paper) of how your arms feel.
6. Wait for a couple of minutes for your arms to feel normal again, shake them a little if necessary.
7. Now let your arms hang down by your sides and imagine a balloon being placed between your arm and rib-cage on each side.
8. Imagine the two balloons being slowly blown up, simultaneously.
9. As the balloons are being blown up they will gently push your arms up.
10. When your arms are level with your shoulders imagine your arms being gently supported by the balloons.
11. Now think of the air being slowly let out of the balloons so that the arms descend gradually down to your sides.
12. Make a note of how your arms feel now, and whether they feel any different from before; if they do you have proved that thought actually does affect functioning because you have performed exactly the same action in each case.

Exercise 2

1. Ask a friend to think of their forehead, then try and push them off balance while they resist.
2. Then do the same thing, only this time ask your friend to think of his (or her) feet being rooted into the ground.
3. Do you experience any difference in the amount of effort that is needed when the person is thinking different thoughts?

Exercise 3

This exercise will clearly demonstrate the power of the mind over the body:

1. Lie down so that you are comfortable. Close your eyes and imagine being in a situation you personally find stressful such as being stuck in the rush-hour when you are late for work or being reprimanded by a figure in authority.
2. After a minute or so notice how your muscles have become tight merely by thinking of the situation.
3. Clear your mind and begin to think of the most pleasant situation you can: perhaps lying on a beach in the Bahamas, or being with your closest friend, or walking in the countryside on a warm summer's day.
4. Again, after a minute or so become aware of how your body has relaxed into a totally different experience from before. You have not even left the room – the cause of the muscular tensing and relaxing took place solely in your mind.

NB It is important to realise that it is essential to have Alexander lessons to experience the directions described in this chapter.

Chapter 11

Senses, Habits and Choices

We can throw away the habit of a lifetime in a few minutes if we use our brains.

FREDERICK MATTHIAS ALEXANDER

At any given moment in our waking life our senses take in information from the outside world to our brain, so that we can make conscious choices. Yet how truly conscious are we about what goes on around us most of the time? We tend to be thinking about what has happened in the past or what may happen in the future. We are rarely in the present. This is because from an early age we are encouraged to think about the future.

While we are thinking of the past or the future we cannot attend to the present – to think about activity. We cannot make conscious choices, and we therefore have to revert to a habitual and automatic mode of behaviour. To practise the Alexander Technique correctly we have to be present and in the here-and-now, in order to make conscious choices in our daily lives. This results in the heightening of our awareness so our senses become more acute.

Exercise

1. Take a walk in the countryside or in a nearby park.
2. Be aware of your sense of sight. For about five minutes look around and see what you can see . . . the trees, the clouds, the grass, and so on.
3. Write down your experience.
4. Then be aware of your sense of hearing . . . what can you

hear? Maybe the wind in the trees, perhaps a child laugh-ing or crying, or the birds singing.
5. Again write down your experiences.
6. Now turn your attention to your sense of smell . . . what can you smell? The flowers, the grass?
7. And now to feeling . . . feel the wind in your hair, the air on your face, or even the breath going in and out of your lungs, and your heart beating in your chest.
8. When you get home, go to the kitchen and make yourself something to eat and focus all your attention on your sense of taste . . . the texture of the food, the flavours, and so on.
9. Take some time to see if you were more aware than you usually are.

If this exercise is performed properly you should see, hear, smell, touch and taste things around you more acutely. We tend to miss a great deal of our lives because we have cultivated this habit of paying too little attention to the present moment. This is to our detriment physically, mentally, emotionally, and spiritually.

Have you ever been on your way to a shop and walked straight past because you were so busy thinking about some-thing else completely? Or driven past your turning and not realized until minutes later? I am sure it happens all the time. Alexander called this 'the mind-wandering habit'.

An old friend and teacher once said, 'The Creator gives man the gift of thought. But what man thinks about is his own gift to himself.' We always have the choice of what to think about, but we usually let our thoughts run wild, and when we do try to exercise some control we find it almost impossible. Giving yourself directions may seem difficult and tedious at first, but I assure you that perseverance will reap great rewards.

HABITS

The dictionary definition of the word 'habit' is:

THE BEHAVIOUR THAT IS GUIDED BY AN AUTOMATIC REACTION TO A SPECIFIC SITUATION.

There are two types of habit to be considered – conscious habits and unconscious habits.

Conscious Habits

These are habits that we are already aware of, such as:

- always sitting in the same chair;
- always having meals at the same time each day;
- smoking;
- drinking;
- cleaning your teeth after every meal;
- biting your finger-nails;
- fidgeting;
- leaving the top off the toothpaste.

Some of these habits are completely harmless, others may even be beneficial, but on the whole, habits tend to be detrimental to a person's natural and spontaneous way of being. By being aware of your habits, you can alter them if you choose.

Unconscious Habits

These are the habits of use to which Alexander constantly referred. These are too numerous to mention, but include:

- stiffening the neck muscles;
- bracing the knees back;
- arching the back in an excessive manner;
- gripping the floor with the toes;
- pushing the hips forward;
- tensing up the shoulders;
- pulling back the head;
- holding the rib-cage rigid.

We all tend unconsciously to have some if not all the above habits, and in order to bring about a desirable change in ourselves we must make conscious that which is unconscious. It is impossible to change a habit while it is still below our level of consciousness. It is vital to recognize the implications of unchecked long-term habits of use on our health and happiness.

In his book *Body Awareness in Action* Professor Frank Pierce Jones writes:

> Habits are not 'an untied bundle' of isolated acts. They interact with one another and together make up an integrated whole.

Whether or not a particular habit is manifest, it is always operative and contributes to character and personality. A man may give himself away in a look or a gesture. A habit cannot be changed without intelligent control of an appropriate means or mechanism. To believe that it can is to believe in magic. People still think, nevertheless, that by passing laws, or by 'wishing hard enough' or 'feeling strongly enough' they can change human behaviour and get a desirable result. That is superstition.

He then goes on to quote the philosopher and writer John Dewey:

The real opposition is not between reason and habit, but between routine or unintelligent habit and intelligent habit or art. Old habits need modification no matter how good they have been. It is the function of intelligence to determine where changes should be made.

Physical, mental and emotional habits

Since the basis of the Alexander Technique rests on the principle that it is impossible to separate the physical, mental and emotional processes in any form of human activity, it follows that any bodily habits we develop in the course of our lives will invariably affect our mental and emotional states. So if indeed you are able to change the way that you perform your physical activities, your mental outlook on life will change, and this in turn will alter how you feel emotionally.

It follows then that feelings of unhappiness or unfulfilment of any kind must of course stem from the way we use our physical bodies, as much as from the way we think with our minds or feel with our emotions. By applying the principles of the Technique (inhibition and direction) a person will invariably alter the way in which they think and feel.

Alexander devotes a whole chapter in his book *Constructive Conscious Control of the Individual* to the subject of happiness, in which he writes:

I shall now endeavour to show that the lack of real happiness manifested by the majority of adults of today is due to the fact that they are experiencing, not an improving, but a continually deteriorating use of their psycho-physical selves. This is associated with those defects, imperfections, undesirable traits of character, disposition, temperament, etc, characteristic of imperfectly co-ordinated people struggling through life beset with certain maladjustments of the psycho-physical organism, which are actually setting up conditions of irritation and pressure during both sleeping and waking hours. Whilst the maladjustments remain present, these malconditions increase day by day and week by week, and foster that unsatisfactory psycho-physical state which we call 'unhappiness'. Small wonder that under these conditions the person concerned becomes more and more irritated and unhappy. Irritation is not compatible with happiness, yet the human creature has to employ this already irritated organism in all the psycho-physical activities demanded by a civilized mode of life. It stands to reason that every effort made by the human creature whose organism is already in an irritated condition must tend to make the creature still more irritated, and therefore as time goes on, his chances of happiness diminish. Furthermore, his experiences of happiness become of ever shorter duration, until at last he is forced to take refuge in a state of unhappiness, a psycho-physical condition as perverted as that state of ill-health which people reach when they experience a perverted form of satisfaction in the suffering of pain.

The psycho-physical condition of the person afflicted with irritation and pressure is such that all his efforts in any direction will be more or less of a failure as compared with the efforts of those who are not so afflicted, and there is probably no stimulus from without which makes more for irritability of the person concerned than failure (either comparative or complete) in accomplishment, nothing which can have a worse effect upon our emotions, self-respect, happiness, or confidence – in fact, upon our temperament and character in general.

In short, the habitual way of being that most of us are encouraged to fall into from childhood onwards, is bound to affect our physical and mental well-being. This in turn will affect our functioning in a detrimental way, which will cause frustration, anger, lack of confidence and a general state of unhappiness. Then these emotional states will themselves start to become habits (see Figs 22 and 23).

No one starts out in life feeling angry or frustrated, no one starts out in life lacking in confidence or lacking in self-worth; these are feelings that we acquire throughout our lives and are not inherent to our mental or emotional make-up.

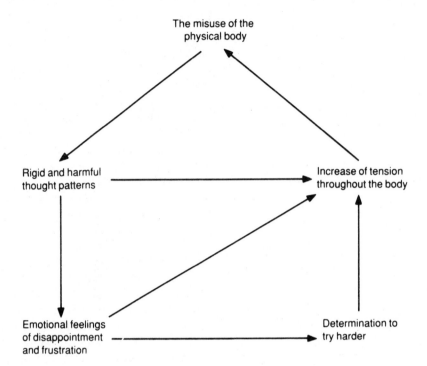

Fig. 22   The perpetual cycle of mental, emotional and physical disharmony.

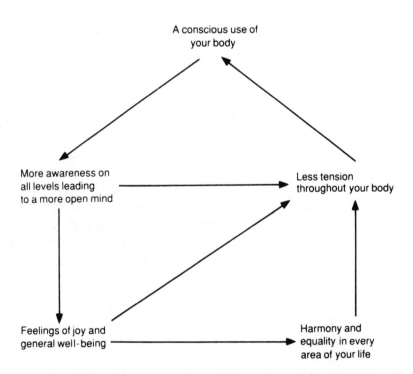

Fig. 23   The perpetual cycle of mental, emotional and physical harmony and well-being.

Exercises

Habits often arise when we are unconscious of the things around us.

Try to be aware of how you normally sit. See if you can notice whether you continually repeat the same positions over and over again. Ask yourself the following questions:

- Do you tend to have your left leg crossed over the right leg, or do you tend to cross your right leg over the left?
- What position do you usually find your feet in?
- What do you do with your arms and hands?
- Do you often have your arms folded or your hands clenched together?
- Have you ever noticed that you sit with your head on one side?

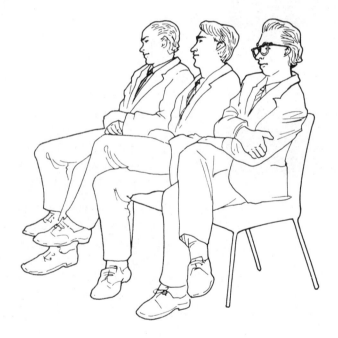

Fig. 24 Adults unknowingly hold tensions in the body even when apparently relaxing. Notice especially the hands and legs.

Even asking yourself these questions will help you to become more aware of certain habits.

To become more aware of your own personal habits also try the following:-

Exercise 1

1. Stand up with your weight evenly distributed on both feet.
2. Now shift the weight on to your right leg by sinking down into your right hip, making sure you do not take your left foot off the ground.
3. Now reverse the procedure bv sinking down into your left hip.
4. Whichever of these two feels more comfortable is your habit.

Exercise 2

Try squeezing a lemon or an orange with the hand you use the least (usually the left hand as most people are right-handed).

Exercise 3

1. Ask a friend to fold their arms; they will probably do this without thinking.
2. Notice which arm is in front of the other.
3. Ask them to fold their arms in the opposite fashion (i.e. the front arm now becomes the back arm).
4. Nine people out of ten find this quite difficult; be sure your friend has in fact folded his arms in the opposite way.

Here is an interesting and true story about the power of habit which happened in the USA not so long ago:

A policeman was waiting at a red light at about 4 am when a car drove through the lights the other way. Because the policeman was feeling drowsy he thought the car had jumped the lights, which of course it had not. He sped after the car with his siren sounding and lights flashing, and eventually pulled the woman driver over. As he was walking to the car he realized to his embarrassment that he had made a mistake. The woman, in a state of panic, and very defensive, said 'What have I done wrong?' The officer, who had become quite sheepish by this point, replied, 'Lady, you just went through a green light.' Because the woman had such a strong habit of being defensive against figures of authority, she responded by saying, 'No, I didn't. No, I didn't. I went through a red light!'

Because our physical habits invariably stem from the rigid way in which we think, with all our preconceived ideas and baseless assumptions, when we become aware and consequently change the patterns of the way in which we move, we are also altering the way in which we think. By understanding and applying those principles underlying the true poise of the body, there are always ways for us to reverse our numerous harmful habits.

CHOICES

> One choice is no choice,
> Two choices is a dilemma,
> Three choices is a real choice.
> *Alan Mars*

There is an old and very wise saying 'When things go wrong, don't go with them.' But this is easier said than done; we have to make a conscious choice about what we are, or are not, going to do at any given moment in time. The freedom to make a real choice in life ultimately leads to the freedom of the spirit which is inherent in each and every one of us. This freedom is essential if man is to regain his dignity and honour which would lead him to reclaiming his rightful place as 'The Crown of Creation'.

One of Alexander's main teachings was that even after making an initial choice we should remain open to 're-choose' at any moment in time.

CHOICE IS: THE POWER TO MAKE A DECISION BASED ON REASON AND DISCRIMINATION RATHER THAN ON FEAR OR HABIT.

I remember very clearly some graffiti written on a wall which stated: 'Two thousand lemmings can't be wrong!' with a picture of lots of lemmings jumping off a cliff.

I also recall a time last summer when I was driving home in heavy holiday traffic. I turned left to go to my home but the car behind me must have thought I knew of a short cut. Many other drivers presumed the same thing until there were eight cars following me. You can imagine their humiliation when I finally parked my car outside my house, which happens to be at the end of a cul-de-sac. An amusing event, but this is how many people operate; tending to do what everyone else is doing instead of thinking for themselves. In a survey of German people, they were asked, 'Why did you personally go to war in 1939?' Nearly all of them said, 'Because everyone else was going – I didn't want to go at all.'

Exercise

This exercise demonstrates the Alexander Technique in a nutshell, but is best done after a few lessons.

1. Choose an action, any one will do, but for the sake of the exercise try raising your arm out in front of you until it is level with your shoulder.
2. Inhibit any immediate response to raise your arm.
3. Give yourself the following instructions or directions:
   (a) Think of your neck being free
   (b) Think of your head going forward and upward
   (c) Think of your back lengthening and widening
4. Continue to project these directions until you believe that you are sufficiently conversant with them to achieve the aim of lifting the arm.
5. While continuing to think of your directions, stop and consciously reconsider your initial decision. Ask yourself whether you will after all go on to perform the action of lifting your arm, or will you not? Or will you do something else altogether such as lifting your leg, for example?
6. Then and there make a fresh decision, either:
   (a) not to go ahead and gain your original 'end', in which case *continue to give yourself* the directions laid down in 3 above;
   or
   (b) to decide to do something different altogether (say, lifting the leg instead of lifting the arm), in which case *continue to give your directions* while you carry out this last decision and actually lift the leg;
   or
   (c) to go ahead after all and lift the arm, in which case *continue to project your directions* to maintain your new 'use' and then perform the action of lifting the arm.

This may seem like a long winded way of going about a simple action, but within this procedure lies the secret of *free choice*.

At first this process may take you some time, but with practice it can be accomplished very swiftly.

In all three cases the essence was to:

STOP

MAKE A DECISION

BUT AT ALL TIMES CONTINUE TO

GIVE YOURSELF THE DIRECTIONS

By sunrise there were nearly a thousand birds standing outside the circle of students, looking curiously at Maynard. They didn't care whether they were seen or not, and they listened, trying to understand Jonathan Seagull. He spoke of very simple things – that it is right for a gull to fly, that freedom is the very nature of his being, that whatever stands against that freedom must be set aside, be it ritual or superstition or limitation in any form.

'Set aside,' came a voice from the multitude, 'even if it be the law of the Flock?'

'The only true law is that which leads to freedom,' Jonathan said. 'There is no other.'

Richard Bach, *Jonathan Livingston Seagull*

Remember: If you do what you have always done ...
You will get what you have always got.

Chapter 12

MUSCLES AND REFLEXES

Everyone wants to be right, but no one stops to consider if their idea of right is right.

FREDERICK MATTHIAS ALEXANDER

The Alexander Technique is a method by which we become more aware of balance, posture and movement in all of our daily activities. Most people have differing ideas about the meaning of the word 'posture'. It is often misinterpreted as 'the way in which we hold ourselves when sitting or standing', but the word hold indicates that we have to 'do' something to ourselves in order to have good posture.

The fact is that there is a complete network of postural muscles throughout our body which can keep us in perfect balance in any given position. In early childhood these muscles help us to keep upright without any effort, but as time goes on we slowly lose the use of these muscles. We then collapse down into ourselves and therefore start to hold ourselves by tensing a completely different set of muscles that are not designed for posture.

MUSCLES

Muscle is the tissue by which, because of its power of contraction, a movement can be initiated or maintained. Since there are over 650 skeletal muscles in the human body muscles are responsible for about 45 per cent of our body weight.

Fig. 25 The surface layer of muscles of the body.

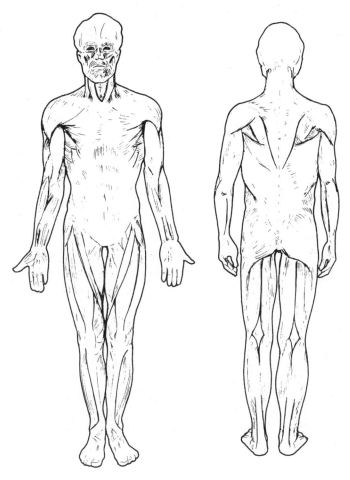

Postural or involuntary muscles

These muscle fibres are so-called because we cannot control them consciously; they work by reflex. They are reddish in colour and never tire when being used. They are some-times known as unstriped muscles from their appearance, and the only function they serve is to keep us upright. They are situated mainly in the torso. The heart muscle, which is involuntary, is partially striped, while certain muscles of the throat and two small muscles inside the ear which are not controllable by will-power are also striped.

The skeletal or voluntary muscles

As the name indicates, these muscle fibres which are white in colour and striped in appearance are almost all attached to the bones of the skeleton. They may have two points of attachment (for example, the biceps joins the shoulder blade to the lower arm or radius); or they may join three bones together (as in the case of the sterno-cleido mastoid which joins the head to the collar bone and the front of the ribcage or sternum).

These muscles vary greatly in size, from the huge gluteus maximus (buttock muscles) to the minute stapedius muscles found in the middle ear.

Voluntary muscles enable us to perform all our actions, both great and small at will. They do this by contracting or relaxing, thus moving the bones to which they are attached. They do, however, tire after a short time. For example, if you hold your arm up for even a few minutes it will begin to ache.

It is easy to see why, if we begin to use our voluntary muscles for posture instead of our involuntary muscles we are going to experience difficulties. The muscles will soon feel tired and either our body will collapse or the muscles become another, possibly leading to one of the common ailments that afflict us.

Muscle contraction

It is important to note that muscles can only pull two bones towards each other, and can never push them apart. This is why they usually work in pairs; one is the prime mover (i.e. the one that is in a state of contraction) and is known as the synergistic muscle; while the other (which slowly relaxes to allow a controlled movement) is called the antagonistic muscle. Obviously all muscles take their turn at being the synergist and then the antagonist. Muscles are in fact pulling against each other all the time, and this is what gives the muscle its tone. The only part of the muscle which does not contract is the connection between bone and the contractile tissue, commonly known as the tendon.

Voluntary muscle movement is controlled by the brain, which co-ordinates all movement using information relayed from the muscle itself, as well as from the eye and the organ of

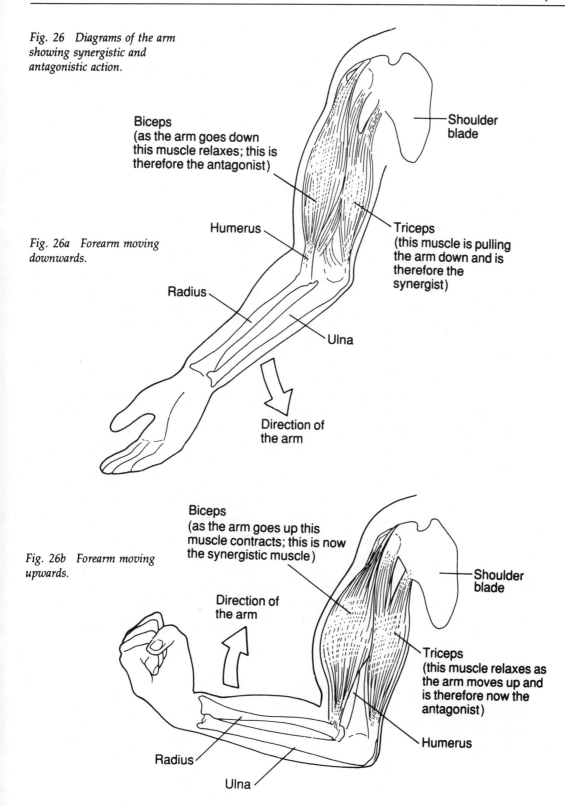

Fig. 26 Diagrams of the arm showing synergistic and antagonistic action.

Biceps
(as the arm goes down this muscle relaxes; this is therefore the antagonist)

Shoulder blade

Humerus

Fig. 26a Forearm moving downwards.

Triceps
(this muscle is pulling the arm down and is therefore the synergist)

Radius

Ulna

Direction of the arm

Biceps
(as the arm goes up this muscle contracts; this is now the synergistic muscle)

Fig. 26b Forearm moving upwards.

Shoulder blade

Direction of the arm

Triceps
(this muscle relaxes as the arm moves up and is therefore now the antagonist)

Humerus

Radius

Ulna

balance situated in the ear. Muscles that require skilled movements, such as those in the hand, have one nerve to only a few fibres, whereas in those that are used for strength (such as gluteus maximus), one nerve will supply a great number of muscle fibres.

How muscles contract

As you can see in Fig. 27 muscles are composed of bundles (fascicles) of muscle cells (or fibres), each enclosed in a partition of fibrous tissue known as the perimysium. These partitions are again surrounded by an outer sheath of tissue known as the fascia (or epimysium). When carefully examined, these bundles of muscle cells, which can be up to twenty centimetres in length, are found to consist of a further collection of fibres which form the units of muscle. It is at this cellular level that the results of practising the Alexander Technique can be discerned.

These fibres (or myofibrils), shorten when chemically activated, which occurs in response to nervous stimulus. The chemical that initiates this depends on the type of muscle, but the response is always the same – namely a shortening of protein molecules.

If muscles are in a constant state of tension, the body will actually remove some of the protein molecules, and this causes a decrease in length of the myofibrils. If this tension persists unchecked it will eventually lead to a shortening of

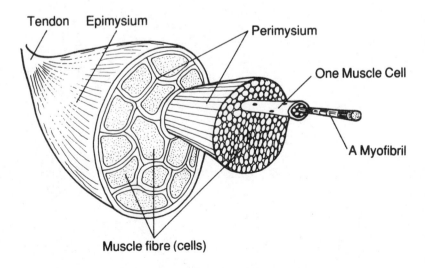

Fig. 27   *The structure of voluntary muscle.*

the whole muscle, as can be illustrated by someone who has one leg shorter than the other, or who in later life has diminished in height.

Thinking of lengthening and widening can bring about a growth in length of the muscle fibres and if this is continued over a period of time the lost protein molecules can be replaced. This in turn will result in an overall lengthening of the muscle or muscles concerned. As I have mentioned before, there are many reports of people who have increased in height by an inch or more during the course of Alexander lessons. But do not worry, this process happens over weeks or months – it is very gradual and gentle!

It is important to note that any excess muscular tension is bound to pull bones out of place (such as a shoulder blade that protrudes rather than rests comfortably on the rib-cage) which will in turn cause other muscles to be unnecessarily taut. So one tense muscle is bound to affect the whole organism.

A prolonged increase in muscle tension will also result in interference in the nervous, digestive, respiratory, and circulatory systems and will inevitably impair natural functions.

THE CIRCULATORY OR VASCULAR SYSTEM

This system consists of arteries, veins and capillaries through which the equivalent of 36,000 litres (8,000 gallons) of blood are pumped every single day. The total length of the blood vessels is an amazing 102,500 kilometres or 64,000 miles, which is half way around the world!

The arteries and veins, like the nerves, weave in and out and between the muscles of the body. They are not rigid tubes, but are able to contract and dilate to let a larger or smaller amount of blood flow through at just the right pressure. If the muscles through which the blood vessels pass are particularly taut, this obviously restricts the flow of the blood, and the heart will then have to work harder to compensate, or parts of the body will be deprived of the nourishment that the blood supplies. This pressure on the arteries and veins can be a major contributing factor in such conditions as varicose veins and even thrombosis.

THE RESPIRATORY SYSTEM

One of the most noticeable things about my students is they have almost all had a habit of shallow breathing; in fact many people only take in about a quarter of the air that a 'normal' breath should supply. The average adult breathes in the region of 13,650 litres (2,800 gallons) of air each day, so it is essential that this system works effectively and efficiently. The reason people suffer from shallow breathing is that they:

- sit in a slumped fashion, which constricts their lung capacity;
- sit in a rigid fashion, so their rib-cage is fixed in one place;
- over-tighten their intercostal muscles (the muscles which connect one rib to another); and
- shorten their back muscles, which in turn causes the rib movement to be restricted.

Exercise

1. Sit in a chair and just notice your breathing: Where are you breathing from? Is your breathing shallow or deep?
2. Now sit in a slumped fashion, the more slumped the better!
3. Take a deep breath and note how much air you are able to take in.
4. This time sit in a very rigid and upright position, as 'straight' as you possibly can.
5. Again take a very deep breath and be aware of how much air is taken in.
6. Lastly sit in a way that is neither slumped nor rigid and take a breath.
7. Compare the three results which should speak for themselves.

From the above exercise it is easy to see that excess muscular activity (or lack of it) will directly affect breathing patterns.

THE DIGESTIVE SYSTEM

The whole digestive system relies heavily on the muscles of the body to perform its natural functions; whether it is the jaw muscles which aid the teeth in chewing food in the first place, or the muscular contractions (peristalsis) that force the food along the digestive tract. In fact the whole of the stomach is a large muscular sac. Since, as I have said before, tension in one muscle will invariably affect the whole muscular system, the free functioning of the processes of digestion, absorption and assimilation will depend on the overall freedom of the entire muscular system.

THE SKELETAL SYSTEM

Bone is a very hard substance indeed, which can last for many centuries so you can imagine the amount of force that the muscles exert when two bones are pulled together and start to wear each other down, as in the case of arthritis.

Because every single bone of the skeleton is inter-connected by the muscles, then if we habitually have excess tension within our structure we are, in reality, pulling one part of ourselves down onto another part. This of course is detrimental to our balance, co-ordination and poise, and eventually to our total well-being, both physical and mental.

THE NERVOUS SYSTEM

The nervous, or neurological, system consists of a network of nerve fibres which run from the brain and the spinal cord (together referred to as the central nervous system), to the rest of the body. The function of this system is to convey messages to and from every part of the organism.

Many of the nerve fibres pass between muscle and bone, as well as between one muscle and another. If a muscle is in a permanent state of contraction due to stress, then the nerves become trapped by the hardened muscle and produce a great deal of pain, such as sciatica. The pain will of course cause the person to tense up even more, thus creating a vicious cycle. Anyone who has experienced a trapped nerve of any description will tell you how painful it is.

Exercise

To demonstrate how hard a muscle may become under tension:

1. Feel your biceps (the muscles of the upper arm) as your arm hangs freely.
2. Pick up a heavy weight such as a chair with only one arm.
3. Note the difference.

REFLEXES

Reflex action is one of the simplest forms of activity of the nervous system. There are three types of reflexes:

Superficial Reflexes
These comprise any sudden movements which result when the skin is lightly brushed or pricked.
Example: The bending movement of the toes when the sole of the foot is stroked firmly from heel to sole.

Deep Reflexes
These are dependent upon the constant state of mild contraction which the muscles are in when at rest.
Example: The patella reflex, more commonly known as the knee-jerk, which occurs when the tendon of the muscle is tapped sharply.

Visceral Reflexes
These are reflexes that are connected with the various organs of the body.
Example: The narrowing of the pupil when a bright light is shone directly into the eye.

All reflex actions occur without any conscious control, yet in some cases they can be overridden by reasoning. If you pick up a hot plate, the reflex action is immediately to drop the plate on to the floor, but our reasoning intelligence knows this will result in a mess on the floor, so the plate is placed down on the table nearby. (This will of course depend on how hot the plate is!) It seems that in animals reflex actions are much more powerful than reasoning. For example, if a cat is chased by a dog it may well run across a busy main road in an attempt to escape, which can lead to tragic consequences. On the contrary, a human being when being chased will sum up the advantages and disadvantages of running out into the road. In this way our rational intelligence can indeed prove sounder than the reflex.

We have reflexes because there are thousands of adjustments that have to be made each minute and we cannot possibly think of them all with our conscious brain. We can, however, still carry out various activities (such as carrying, bending, walking or reaching out) that, by rights, should upset our balance and cause us to topple over, if it were not for our muscular system making continuous adjustments of tension and position through our reflexes.

Here are four examples of how the use or misuse of ourselves can affect some of the major reflexes:

The 'falling' reflex

Whenever our structure is off-balance and likely to fall backwards, a fear reflex, situated in and around the neck area, comes into play. This is not unlike 'the startle pattern' which

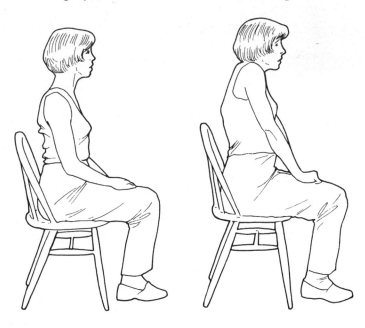

Fig. 28   The fear reflex.

Fig. 28a   Normal shoulder position.

Fig. 28b   The fear reflex.

a   b

is brought about by a sudden noise. It is interesting to observe that this behaviour may appear in the neck muscles and nowhere else. The head is pulled backwards as the muscles shorten and the shoulders become hunched, the very actions recognized by Alexander as being habits common to all humans. There is good reason for this response to falling backwards; it protects the lower parts of the brain, the cerebellum and the medulla, as well as the top of the spinal cord. Any damage to these areas would render a person incapacitated for life. Most of us, however, trigger this reflex every time we sit down in a chair, because in order to sit we tend to fall back for at least part of the way.

Exercise

1. Place your hands so that they rest on the back of the neck with the middle fingers just touching.
2. Stand with your back to a sofa as though you were about to sit down.
3. Now sit down by falling backwards, while trying to notice any pressure on your hands.

It is likely that you felt your neck muscles stiffen in the process – this is the fear reflex which is often unnecessarily activated every time we sit or stand, until it becomes a constant habit.

The knee reflex

This is perhaps the most well-known reflex in the body. Doctors use it to test the reflex system by tapping gently on the tendon just below the patella (kneecap). This reflex aids in walking. The lower leg muscles of the leg behind the leading one are stretched over the patella; this activates the reflex so the leg will 'kick' into the next step.

The postural reflexes

Recent experiments by Dr David Garlick, a senior lecturer in physiology at the University of New South Wales in Sydney, have shown that many of the postural muscles in the torso are activated by sensory nerve endings in the feet. These nerve endings are sensitive to pressure, so the more weight there is on our feet the better the postural muscles will work. (This happens even when sitting down if the soles of the feet are on the ground – though obviously not to the same extent.) However, as I have said before, many people do not position their feet correctly when they stand; they tend to put too much weight on either their heels or their toes, or alternatively put most of their weight on one side.

In such cases, the sensory nerve endings cannot be stimulated, and there will be no activation of the postural muscles which automatically keep us erect. As a result, we start to use our skeletal muscles instead, and because they tire very quickly we inevitably begin to slump.

Re-education, using the principles of the Technique, can start to restore the body's rightful balance, thus encouraging the appropriate muscles to be used for the appropriate purpose.

The toe reflexes

Between the metatarsal bones of the foot, which end as the five toes, there are four sets of muscles called the dorsal interossei. Attached to each of these muscles there are sensory nerve endings which activate the muscles of the leg. Like the postural reflexes, these operate mainly when standing. If, as before, we are not standing evenly on our feet, these reflexes will not work effectively and once again we will have to involve our voluntary system which requires much more effort.

Exercise

You can test this reflex very easily for yourself:

1. Ask a friend to sit in a chair.
2. Make sure they are sitting erect. Place a hand on their knee and move their leg from side to side. It should move quite easily.
3. Now ask them to lean forward so more of their weight is on their feet and less on their sitting bones.
4. Again place your hand on their knee, and try to move their leg from side to side once again. This time the leg should not move so easily.

Because more weight is on the toes, the nerve endings between the toes are activated, causing the leg muscles to tighten, ready for the standing position.

> Mr. Alexander's method lays hold of the individual as a whole, as a self-vitalizing agent. He reconditions and re-educates the reflex mechanisms and brings their habits into normal relation with the functioning of the organism as a whole. I regard this method as thoroughly scientific and educationally sound.
>
> *Prof. George E. Coghill, anatomist and physiologist*

Stretch reflexes in connection with the Alexander Technique

A stretch reflex is the response of a muscle which contracts when it is stretched. The stretch may be caused by a stimulus such as the upward pressure of the intervertebral discs of the spine, or by an external force such as gravity. The function of the stretch reflex is to stop one part of the body dislocating from the rest of the structure if it is suddenly or unexpectedly pulled – like the inertia-reel seat belts used in most cars today.

In other words, if an arm is pulled to try and make it longer, the effect will in fact be to shorten the arm still further. This begs the question whether traction can in some cases cause a shortening of the structure. Professor Frank Pierce Jones writes:

> The tendency of the body to lengthen from within gives it strength as well as buoyancy. If the discs have expanded, the small muscles attached to the vertebrae must have been lengthened and their strength thereby increased. The lengthening and strengthening initiated by the discs and the small muscles would be transmitted by purely mechanical means to the longer muscles and the process would continue to the surface. This lengthening–strengthening process is further enhanced by movement. In moving the body or one of its parts against gravity the lifting muscles are facilitated by the stretch placed upon them by the part that is being lifted (a movement against gravity is facilitated by gravity itself). In getting up from a chair, for example, the head, neck, and back move forward as a unit without losing their length. In the process the muscles in the lower back, buttocks, and thighs are stretched. When the stretch reaches a certain level of intensity, the stretched muscles contract reflexly, straightening the hip joint and in turn stretching the muscles around the knee. The body is thus lifted smoothly and easily with a sense of little or no effort.

This is the sort of experience a pupil has during an Alexander lesson, referred to as 'the Alexander experience'.

Exercise

1. Sit on a kitchen chair.
2. Stand up in your normal way.
3. Sit down again, in your usual manner.
4. Now stand up again, but this time move your torso in one piece from the hips, with a sense of slightly falling forward out of the chair.
5. Sit down, again think about bending forwards from the hips with a sense of falling forward.

Try this a few times and you will begin to see how new ways of standing up and sitting down can be done with much less effort.

Exercise

Most people try to improve their posture with their voluntary muscles instead of their postural muscles. Since the voluntary muscles tire easily you can see whether you are also using the wrong muscles to improve your posture.

1. Stand or sit in front of a mirror as before.
2. See if you can notice anything about your posture that you would like to change.
3. If you can, put yourself into a position that you are happy with.
4. Wait for a few minutes so that you can see whether your muscles begin to tire. If they do, you know that you have increased muscular tension to improve your posture instead of releasing it.

Chapter 13

MEANS AND ENDS

Until one is committed there is hesitancy, the chance to draw back, always ineffectiveness. Concerning all acts of Initiative and Creation, there is one elementary truth, the ignorance of which kills countless ideas and splendid plans, that the moment one definitely commits oneself, then Providence moves too. All sorts of things occur to help one that would never have occurred. A whole stream of events issues from the decision, raising in one's favour all manner of unforeseen incidents and material assistance which no man could have dreamed would have come his way.

W. H. MURRAY

Whatever you can do or think you can, begin it. Boldness has Genius, Power and Magic in it. Begin it now.

GOETHE

END-GAINING

What Alexander called 'end-gaining', we today call 'goal-orientation'. This is the fundamental approach of our educational system.

Give a child conscious control and you give him poise, the essential starting point for education. Without that poise, which is a result aimed at by neither the old nor the new methods of education, he will presently be cramped and distorted by his environment.

Frederick Matthias Alexander

The end-gaining approach which we are taught at school seems to permeate every sphere of life. As a race, we are and always have been trying to make our life more comfortable and enjoyable. This is only natural. Yet surely it is just as natural to look at the consequences of the actions that bring about this desired end; in other words, to attend to the 'means whereby' such an end can come about. When we fail to do so we are often cutting down the branch on which we are sitting. Just consider for a moment the incredible amount of pollution that we create on the planet every single day.

Back in 1968 I remember a 'Horizon' programme called 'Owing To Lack Of Consideration Tomorrow Has Been Cancelled'. That was over twenty years ago; yet it is only recently that people have begun to be aware of the effect pollution is having on our planet. We go on making the same mistakes over and over again, even though the results of our actions are pointed out so clearly. We can see this clearly in the 'Greenhouse Effect' which is threatening every species on the planet, including ourselves.

Is it not strange that man has become so skilled in the nature and workings of the machines he has created and yet knows so little about the mechanisms of his own organism? Alexander wrote in his last book:

> Man knows all about the means whereby he can keep the in-animate machine in order, and considers it his duty to make proper use of these, but he knows little or nothing about the means whereby he can keep in order that animate human machine – himself. The great majority of people have not yet awakened to the great and growing need of such a 'means whereby' and so have not yet appreciated that these are essential to the art of living healthily, happily and in harmony with one another.

The means whereby

It is of course, necessary for us to have goals in life, and to attain them; this is only human. It is what we do to ourselves and others in the process that we need to look at. The way we go about our everyday activities is a reflection of what we do to our planet; after all if we do not respect ourselves how are we ever going to respect the planet on which we live? Attending to the means whereby an end is attained is simply a case of stopping for a moment and thinking things through to their natural conclusion.

Trying to gain an end without thinking of the best way for

that end to be attained can become a habit – a habit of living in the future. Achieving a goal by considering each step of the way in a conscious manner encourages us to remain in the present, and as a result we are far more likely to achieve the end that we set out to accomplish.

Attending to the 'means whereby' does not mean being over-careful or cautious; it means applying common sense to any given situation.

Trying

When you think carefully about the way in which actions are performed, the old saying: 'When at first you don't succeed, try, try, and try again' becomes: 'When at first you don't succeed, never try again . . . At least not in the same way.'

Trying invariably involves excessive and unnecessary tension. It was not until Alexander gave up trying that he achieved the end he had been trying to reach for many years, namely to stop pulling his head back when he talked.

Exercises

It is very simple, what is meant by ends and means:

1. Find yourself a spacious area such as a large room or, better still, the garden.
2. Be at one end of the room or garden and choose an object at the other end, and without thinking go and touch that object.
3. Repeat the same procedure, only this time before you walk to the object, decide how you are going to reach that object.
4. Repeat this process several times choosing a different way each time.

The first way would be your habitual way, with no conscious means applied, but the other ways, of which there are thousands, were performed by a conscious 'means whereby'.

When I have given this exercise at my evening classes it is surprising how many people cannot think of more than three or four ways of achieving their goal.

If you have the same problem here are a few different ways you can use:

Running
Walking
Crawling
Hopping
Skipping
Tip-toeing
Stomping
Jumping
Wriggling on your tummy.

Then if you take walking for instance, there are so many different ways in which you can walk:

Fast
Medium
Slow
  (with many variations in between)
In a straight line
In an arc
In a zig-zag
Forwards
Backwards
Sideways
While leaning sideways
While leaning backwards
While leaning forwards
While twisting from side to side.

You can of course combine one or more of the above; for example you could tip-toe slowly sideways, but in a straight line, while you are slightly leaning forwards! The combinations are endless.

Another exercise is to think of a completely different way of moving that is not mentioned above. If you want to watch an expert just watch a young child, and you will be amazed how often they change their style of moving. One moment they are walking, the next they are skipping, then they run for a few steps and so on.

Take walking once again: See how many different ways you can think of getting from 'A' to 'B'. Enjoy finding the many thousands of possible ways that your body has of moving.

At first you may quickly run out of ideas, but when you become more experienced there is a wide range of ways in which you can move.

The problem for us all, is that in order to be more conscious, we have to start living in a new way. The principles of inhibition and direction must be applied, instead of the hazardous end-gaining behaviour of the past. Like everything else in nature, this is a slow process and we must be content with a steady progress from day to day. It is easy to become anxious about being on the right track, even though we know now that what we perceive as right is so often wrong. However, with patience you will continue to improve as you consciously attend to the means whereby you perform your day-to-day activities.

Chapter 14

Give Your Back a Rest

*A perfect spine is an all-important factor in preserving those
conditions and uses of the human machine which work together
for perfect health, yet there are comparatively few people who do
not in some form or degree suffer, perhaps quite unconsciously,
from spinal curvature.*

FREDERICK MATTHIAS ALEXANDER

THE SPINE

The spine, also known as the vertebral column or the back-
bone, forms an important part of the skeleton. It acts both as a
pillar which supports the upper parts of the body, and as a
protection to the spinal cord and the nerves which arise from
it. The spinal column is built up of a number of bones placed
one upon another; these are called the vertebrae. The presence of a spinal cord which is supported by a vertebral
column in more evolved types of animal gives them the title of
vertebrates, and of all the vertebrates it is only man who can
stand absolutely erect. This, besides having distinct advantages, brings with it certain problems, the main one being that
gravity is now bearing down upon a structure that is
extremely unstable because it has two legs instead of four.

The spine is about 28 inches (70 centimetres) long in a fully
grown adult. Differences in height mainly depend upon the
length of the lower limbs. There are thirty-three vertebrae
which make up the complete spinal column, although in
adults five of these are fused together to form the sacrum, and
a further four to form the coccyx; the actual number of separate bones is therefore reduced to twenty-six. Of these, there
are seven in the neck area which are referred to as the cervical

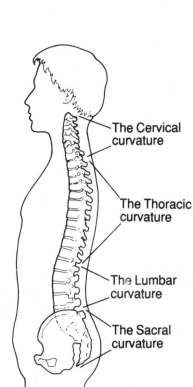

Fig. 29 Diagram of the spine showing the four curves.

The Cervical curvature

The Thoracic curvature

The Lumbar curvature

The Sacral curvature

vertebrae; twelve below these which all have ribs attached and are known as the thoracic or dorsal vertebrae; a further five below these which are called the lumbar vertebrae; and lastly the nine which go to make up the sacrum and coccyx.

An important feature of the spine, especially marked in human beings, is the presence of four curves. These curves strengthen the structure so that it can bear more weight, and they also act as a spring to minimize any jolting or jarring of the internal organs. If the curves become too straight, or more often too pronounced, the spine will lose some of these properties; that is, it will become weaker and will not suspend and support the organs as efficiently as it should.

Intervertebral discs

Between each vertebra lies a thick layer of fibro-cartilage known as the intervertebral disc. Each disc consists of an outer portion, which is known as the annulus fibrosus, and an inner core known as the nucleus pulposus.

The annulus fibrosus

This part of the disc is made up of concentric fibres which keep the nucleus in place when it is under pressure from above.

The nucleus pulposus

This central part of the disc consists of a gelatinous substance which is transparent. It is in fact made up of 88 per cent water and it is this nucleus that takes the brunt of the body's weight (*see* Fig. 31).

BACK PAIN

There are many types of backache: sciatica, lumbago or a slipped disc, to name a few. The majority of painful backs stem from mechanical or structural disorders which directly result from constant misuse of the body. Moving habitually in a way that puts enormous strain on the spine causes the

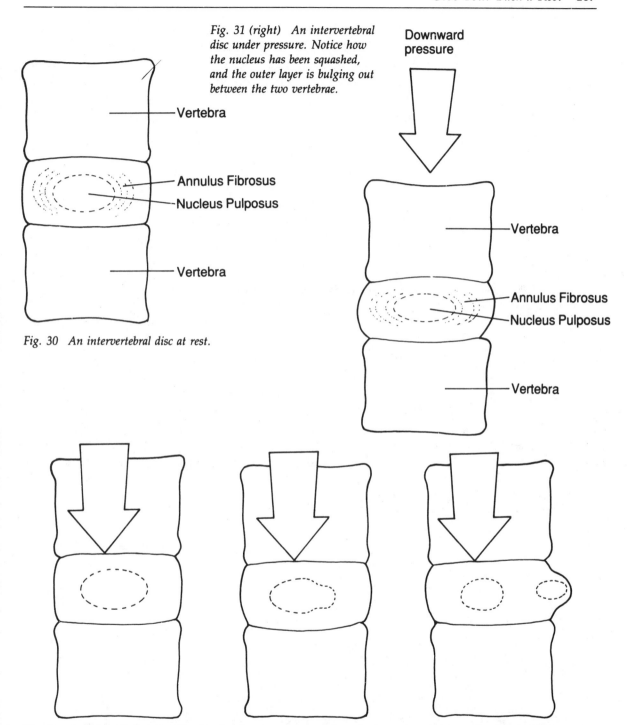

Fig. 31 (right) An intervertebral disc under pressure. Notice how the nucleus has been squashed, and the outer layer is bulging out between the two vertebrae.

Downward pressure

Vertebra

Annulus Fibrosus
Nucleus Pulposus

Vertebra

Vertebra

Annulus Fibrosus
Nucleus Pulposus

Vertebra

Fig. 30 An intervertebral disc at rest.

Fig. 32 A prolapsed disc. Prolonged and unequal pressure on the spine can cause the disc to be squashed between the adjacent vertebrae. This can cause the nucleus of a disc to be split in half, and one of the halves can make its way to the edge of the outer layer, thus coming into contact with a nerve. This naturally gives rise to great pain.

nucleus of the disc to be squashed between the two vertebrae (*see* Fig. 32). Nerves can become trapped between the vertebrae as in the case of sciatica, or the nucleus can come under such pressure that it is forced through the layer of annulus fibrosus, thus rupturing the outside membrane. This of course is extremely painful, as anyone who has suffered from a prolapsed disc (slipped disc) will tell you.

There is one position which will take all pressure off the spine, and ease any pain in the lumbar region (the most common site of back pain), and which will prevent you suffering from backache in the future. This position is called the *semi-supine position*, the word 'supine' simply meaning 'lying face up'.

The Semi-Supine Position

This exercise is often considered the hallmark of the Alexander Technique. It is simply to lie down on your back with some books underneath your head, your knees bent, your feet flat on the floor, and your hands resting gently on either side of your navel (*see* Fig. 33). The number of books beneath the head will vary from person to person, and in some cases from day to day. The best way to find out the right amount is simply to ask your teacher when you start having Alexander lessons. As a rough guide, follow these instructions:

Fig. 33   The semi-supine position is especially good for lower back pain.

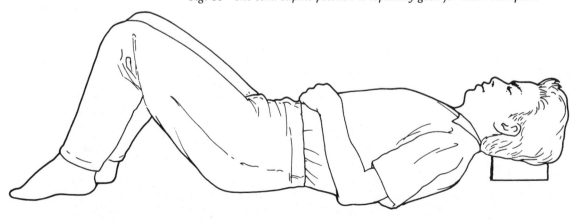

1. Stand against a flat surface such as a door.
2. Just stand in your normal way (do not try to stand up straight) with your buttocks and shoulder-blades just touching the door.
3. Get a friend or relative to measure the distance between the door and the back of your head.
4. To this measurement add one inch, and this should be roughly the height of books you need.

Remember: it is better to have too many books beneath your head than too few, but make sure there is no restriction whatsoever to your breathing.

The reason you have the books underneath the head is to give it support and to help combat the habit of pulling the head back. It should be noted, however, that it is still possible to pull your head back on to the books when you are simply lying there.

The soles of your feet should have as much contact with the ground as possible, with the knees pointing to the ceiling. The feet should be as near to your buttocks as is comfortably possible. The legs may well want to fall in towards each other, or out away from each other. If this is so follow one of these instructions:

1. *If the legs fall inwards* then move the feet closer together.
2. *If the legs fall outwards* then move the feet further away from each other.

This will reduce muscle tension in the legs to the absolute minimum.

The back should be in as much contact with the ground as possible, but be sure not to *do* anything in order to flatten it. The reason the knees are raised is to enable the lower back to release on to the floor in comfort.

As most of us have rounded shoulders, the hands rest on the abdomen so that the shoulders can release backwards.

Try and give yourself at least twenty minutes a day to lie in this position. At first lie for five minutes only and then add on another minute each day, until you have built up to twenty minutes. While you are on the floor give yourself the following directions:

• Allow the neck to be free.
• Think of the head going forward and up (but don't forget

this is in relation to the spine and *not* in relation to the floor).
- Allow the back to lengthen and widen.
- Think of the shoulders widening.
- Think of the knees pointing up to the ceiling.

As you are lying there try also to be aware of any specific tension you may be holding and just let it go. It is also useful and interesting to be aware of your breathing. Ask yourself:

- Where do I feel any movement?
- How deeply am I breathing?
- Is my rib-cage moving?
- How fast am I breathing?

Remember, as I have said before, that real and lasting change is a slow process, so persevere and be patient. Make notes each time.

SOME INTERESTING FACTS ABOUT THE SPINE

Our height changes between the morning and the evening. We can lose as much as an inch or more during a day, but we regain this while we are sleeping at night. I once had a pupil, a midwife, who was a little on the short side. She consciously arranged any job interviews as early in the morning as possible; so she would appear taller!

During the 1930s a physician from Budapest, named DePuky, measured the heights of 1,216 people between the ages of five and ninety (a) just before they got out of bed in the morning, and (b) just before they went to bed at night. He found there was an increase in height in the morning averaging 1.61 centimetres; that is, approximately one per cent of the body's height.

The main reason for this change was the size and shape of the intervertebral discs which lost fluid during the day while the spine was under pressure, and regained it at night when the spine was horizontal. A large percentage of this fluid is regained within the first twenty minutes of lying down. This is why lying down in the middle of the day regenerates the discs so they can work more effectively and efficiently for the rest of the day.

THE DECLINE OF MAN'S STATURE WITH AGE

Have you ever noticed that your parents or grandparents seem to 'shrink' with age? Well the fact is, they do. A scientist named Junghanns performed 1,142 postmortem dissections of the spinal column, and found that the ratio between the thickness of the discs and the thickness of the adjacent vertebrae diminished with age:

- At birth they were the same size;
- at ten the disc was half the size of the vertebra;
- at twenty-four the disc was a third of the size of the vertebra;
- at sixty the disc was a quarter of the size of the vertebra.

Up to the age of twenty the bones are still growing so some of these figures are not surprising. But after the early twenties there is no reason for the discs to diminish in size apart from the excess pressure that is placed on them by continuous muscular tension. This pressure causes a gradual loss of fluid from the fibro-cartilage of which the discs are largely composed. The spine is a hydraulic system which works by absorbing and releasing water; it can in fact absorb up to twenty times its volume of water. You can see that if the discs have shrunk in size then the spine cannot work to its maximum capability.

If you lie down regularly each day for a mere twenty minutes then not only are you easing or preventing backache, but you will be ensuring that the discs in your back are able to maintain their correct shape for longer. This will give you the chance to move in a more effortless way.

Exercise

1. Observe yourself while standing side-on in front of a mirror. Notice particularly the curves in your back.
2. Lie down for twenty minutes.
3. Stand in front of the mirror once again and see if you can notice any difference.

The way in which you go into and come out of the semi-supine position is also very important. Figure 34 will help you to get the most out of your session.

Getting into and coming out of the semi-supine position

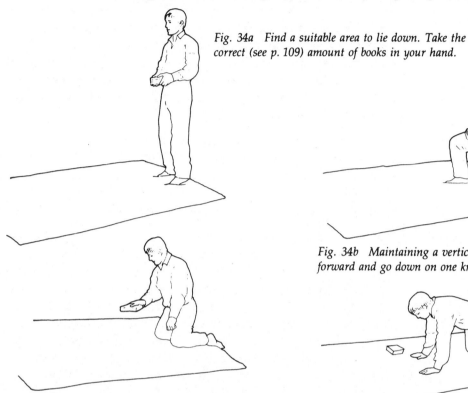

Fig. 34a   Find a suitable area to lie down. Take the correct (see p. 109) amount of books in your hand.

Fig. 34b   Maintaining a vertical torso put one leg forward and go down on one knee.

Fig. 34c   Place the books to your right or left, roughly where your head will be when you are lying down.

Fig. 34d   Place your hands on the ground so that you are on all fours.

Fig. 34e   Lift yourself up so that you are balanced on your hands and toes.

Fig. 34f   Lower your legs to the ground with your knees pointing in the opposite direction to the books.

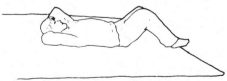

Fig. 34g   Gently roll over on to your back, adjusting the position of the books so that they are comfortably under the back of your head.

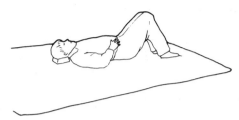

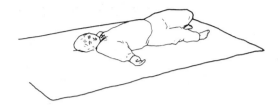

Fig. 34h   Bring your knees upwards positioning your feet so that they are as near as possible to your torso while still remaining comfortable.
Decide which way you wish to get up. Look in that direction and then let your knees roll in that direction.

Fig. 34i   After lying down for twenty minutes or so, take a few moments to think about how you can get up while still maintaining the length in your spine.

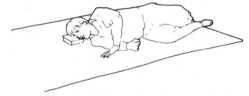

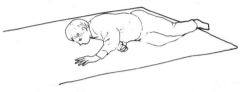

Fig. 34j   Let your whole body roll off the books.

Fig. 34k   Roll over on to your front with the support of a hand and a leg.

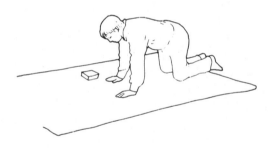

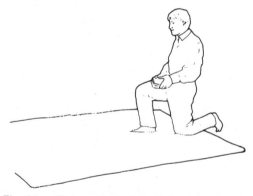

Fig. 34l   Raise yourself until you are on all fours once again.

Fig. 34m   Pick up the books and then place one leg in front of the other.

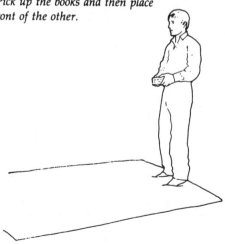

Fig. 34n   Thinking of the head going forward and up, lean forward and you will naturally come back to the standing position. Note that this is only one of many ways of getting up, but it is useful to start with. It is also valuable to learn to follow a given set of instructions as this will reveal your habits. Experiment with rolling on to different sides while getting up and down.

Chapter 15

What to Expect from an Alexander Lesson

All I need say in this place is that I am sure, as a matter of personal experience and observation, that it gives all the things we have been looking for in a system of physical education: relief from strain due to maladjustment, and consequent improvement in physical and mental health; increased consciousness of the physical means employed to gain the end proposed by the will and, along with this a general heightening of consciousness on all levels; a technique of inhibition, working on the physical level to prevent the body from slipping back, under the influence of greedy 'end-gaining', into its old habits of mal-coordination, and working to inhibit undesirable impulses and irrelevance on the emotional and intellectual levels respectively. We cannot ask more from any system of physical education; nor if we seriously desire to alter human beings in a desirable direction, can we ask any less?

ALDOUS HUXLEY, *Ends and Means*

INDIVIDUAL LESSONS

This is clearly the best way to find out more about yourself. A lesson will last between thirty and forty-five minutes, and the aims of the lessons are:–

- To detect any tension that you may be holding unnecessarily and then to release it.
- To become aware of the habits of mind–body use that are causing the tension, and to change these if you so wish.
- To develop different ways of performing actions which will not create so much tension in the first place.
- To teach you inhibition and apply directions.
- To give you an experience of an improved use of yourself.

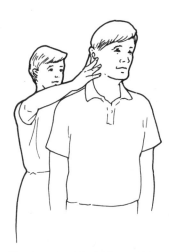

Fig. 35 An Alexander teacher works with her pupil to release tension and achieve a free, dynamic relationship of the head, neck and upper back.

The role of the teacher

The teacher's role is to point out your own personal habits, and explain why they are so harmful. He or she will give certain directions to help you combat your old ways of moving. This is done through verbal instructions and also by use of the hands, much of which is carried out around the head, neck and back area. The touch of the hands is very subtle indeed, and will not aggravate any pain. However, if you are suffering a great deal it may be advisable to obtain treatment (from your doctor, chiropractor or osteopath) before going for lessons.

The teacher may also work with you on a table at first. (Note you will not be required to remove your clothes – except perhaps your shoes.) In this position, gravity affects you least, and it will therefore be easier for you to release tension.

After this you may be taken through a series of movements, such as sitting or walking, so that you can learn different ways of moving. If any of these activities should cause you discomfort or pain, your teacher will be happy to review these with you to shed light on the cause. Occasionally you may experience an extra ache or tension; this is probably due to muscle lengthening and is no cause for concern. It is similar to the 'growing pains' you felt as a child, and should not last more

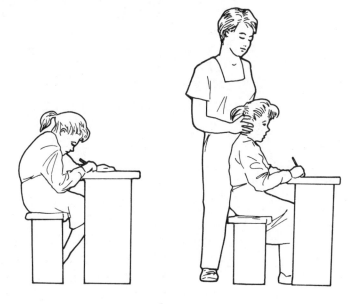

Fig. 36 Many years of hunching over school work can seriously affect our posture and breathing later in life. An Alexander teacher can help us to perform regular activities such as this in a new and improved way.

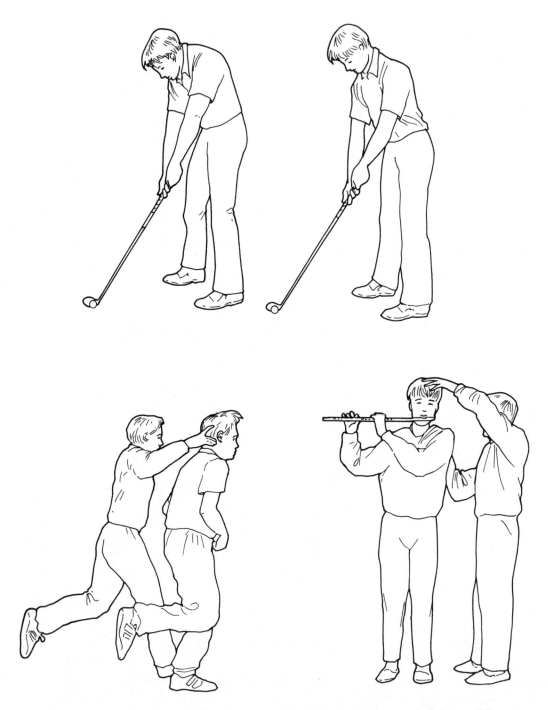

Fig. 37 *Alexander lessons can be applied to practically any activity.*

than a few hours. In the end an Alexander Lesson can be applied to almost any activity (*see* Fig. 37).

The number of lessons needed will vary from person to person, but the changes will be noticeable from the first lesson.

The price of lessons also varies a great deal, depending on the experience of the teacher, and the particular part of the country. They can range from as little as £8.00 to more than £20.00 per lesson. Some people are put off by the price of a course of lessons, but it is worth considering that the cost is less than an average holiday and the effects will last long after your holiday is only a distant memory. It is a matter of priorities; this could be essential for your future well-being. If you really cannot afford a full course of lessons then three or four will definitely be of help, but you should discuss this with your teacher before you start.

It is strongly recommended to try one lesson from a variety of teachers because a good rapport with a certain teacher will greatly enhance the process of change.

There is a list of Alexander Technique Societies worldwide at the back of this book. You can apply to them for names of teachers who have trained on courses authorized by the Society of Teachers of the Alexander Technique (STAT).

LEARNING IN GROUPS

It is also of great value to participate in classes in the Technique. These are often organized by local adult education authorities. Even if you are already having private lessons, group sessions can be revealing too. It is easier to perceive misuse in someone else when they are performing simple acts like sitting down or standing up, and most of us share the same habits. By watching other people you can make comparisons and see exactly what you are doing. You then have the choice of whether or not to change your unconscious behaviour patterns.

These group classes are not expensive: around £2.50 for a two-hour session. I have been amazed at the physical changes I have seen in people who come to these classes, and by the noticeable difference in their outlook on life.

Whether you have private lessons or learn in a group situation, I reiterate my point that your current habits will *feel right* and a new use of yourself is therefore bound to feel very alien. This feeling is only temporary. Within a few weeks the new way of moving will begin to feel natural and your old habits will feel clumsy and awkward. You have to approach it with the idea of *unlearning*, rather than learning something new.

You must be prepared to be told where you are going wrong, and this is something none of us likes. The irony is that as we progress we will be improving our use of ourselves but we will not know it – and neither will we want to! As Alexander once said:

> The right thing to do would be the last thing we should do, left to ourselves, because it would be the last thing we should think it would be the right thing to do.

THE PHYSICAL BENEFITS

Any pain you may be feeling due to mal-co-ordination or tension throughout the muscular system, will slowly but surely begin to diminish. The intensity of the pain will start to abate, and the intervals between the bouts of pain will gradually lengthen. This may take some time but, unlike many other forms of treatment, the effects of Alexander lessons are permanent.

It is important to understand, however, that you have a definite part to play; the teacher can only help. It is you who has to make the deliberate and reasoned decision to alter your way of being. This is why the Alexander Technique is never heralded as a cure or remedy; the only person who brings about a cure is you yourself – you have only to be taught how to do it.

The effect of a lesson is to experience lightness and ease within your body, and a sense of being generally more in touch with your body. This effect will last only a short time at first, but will gradually increase as your lessons progress. Eventually you will be able to retain this feeling of well-being between lessons, and it is then that you may reduce the frequency of your lessons.

Many people report sensations of 'floating down the street', movements start to become effortless and generally people start to move through life with much greater ease.

THE EMOTIONAL BENEFITS

The sensation of physical lightness that we experience has a profound effect on how we feel emotionally. Pupils who have been highly-strung or anxious begin to feel calmer; those who have been depressed start to feel brighter and realize that life isn't quite so bad after all. People on the whole begin to feel happier within themselves which of course rubs off on people around them and consequently has many repercussions in their lives.

It should be remembered, however, that any emotion suppressed for a long time may emerge, and this may be a little uncomfortable for a short while. The most common emotions to be suppressed are anger and sadness, and you may indeed start to experience these at the slightest thing. This is a normal part of the process and will quickly pass. If necessary, discuss any emotional changes with your teacher, for they will be more than happy to reassure you.

Generally however, it is the positive emotions – happiness, joy, contentment, freedom – that have been repressed, and it is these that start to surface. When this happens we can begin to reduce feelings of unhappiness, misery, sadness and gloom from our lives.

THE MENTAL BENEFITS

Because the result of a lesson is to feel much calmer, we will be able to think more clearly about the decisions we have to make in life. We will actually have more time to think about these things and thus be more likely to make the correct choices from day to day. Making the right decisions will naturally make us feel better about ourselves. In short, we become a more reasonable and clear-thinking human being; our self-esteem is boosted, and our self-confidence improves.

THE SPIRITUAL BENEFITS

When you feel emotionally calmer, mentally more balanced, and physically lighter you can more easily begin to experience your spirit – the joy of existence. Many people have this feeling as a child, but tend to lose it as they become involved in the superficialities of present-day living. Alexander lessons will help the chains of our rigid thought patterns fall away, to reveal a being that we had forgotten existed. We can begin to feel a deep peace and inner freedom ... we start to feel who we really are. Alexander called this our 'Supreme Inheritance'.

> The physical, mental and spiritual potentialities of the human being are greater than we have ever realised, greater perhaps than the human mind in its present evolutionary stage is capable of realising.
>
>   We must break the chains which have so held us to that direct-ive mental plane which belongs to the early stages of his evolu-tion. The adoption of conscious guidance and control, which is man's supreme inheritance, must follow, and the outcome will be a race of men and women who will outstrip their ancestors in every known sphere, and enter new spheres as yet undreamt of by the great majority of the civilized peoples of our time.
>
>   *Frederick Matthias Alexander*

So, the question is not whether you can afford to take Alexander lessons, but rather, can you afford not to?

Chapter 16

Case Histories

What would you attempt to do if you knew you could not fail.
DR ROBERT SCHULLER

This chapter is made up of contributions from various people who have had experience of the Alexander Technique. In their own words they describe the difference it has made to their lives.

CASE HISTORY
Christine Mills
Age: Thirty-seven
Occupation:
Teacher/housewife

Last September, my five-year-old son started school. After a few days of feeling lost and a little sad, I began to experience a sense of emancipation – no ties and a whole world of new activities in which to become involved. During the last five years I had taken an interest in alternative medicine as my son was a chronic sufferer of asthma and eczema. Homoeopathy had become important in our lives as it had completely cured both of these illnesses.

Since then other therapies have continued to interest me, so when I discovered an evening class entitled 'Posture and Pain' I decided to enrol. I had heard that it had something to do with relieving tension and back pain, and as a pianist this was enough to make me interested in finding out more. I was, however, totally unprepared for the way in which its philosophy would revolutionize my life and my being.

Later that September, having embarked upon my new interests, I discovered that I was pregnant. I was not overjoyed, more dismayed, because my new-found freedom was about to disappear and the prospect of childbirth filled me with dread. After a few weeks of soul searching I began to feel that here was a chance for me to get it right this time and to enjoy the previously denied pleasures of pregnancy, childbirth and babyhood. Certain aspects of the Alexander Technique helped me to maintain this positive attitude.

One of the most important aspects of the course for me was the concept of being aware of the here-and-now. I have always been one to dwell in the past and to look forward to the future, often with apprehension. In fact I am a habitual day-dreamer. I began to enjoy the pregnancy itself and stopped worrying about the future or the past. I began to have times when I could draw into myself and enjoy simply being, particularly during the twenty minutes per day we were advised to spend on our backs letting go of the tension in our muscles. During these times I was able to come to terms with my fear of childbirth which had remained with me since the traumatic birth of my son five years before.

In fact, fear, and dealing with this most destructive of emotions, was one of the issues that came up during our course. I realised that fear and ignorance go hand in hand, so I became determined to become as informed as possible about pregnancy, physiology and childbirth. I began to realize why my last experience had been so needlessly traumatic and painful, and I began to prepare for the ideal birth – at home. Many people tried to dissuade me but for the first time in my life I was developing an inner confidence that, on this matter at least, was unshakeable.

Among other aspects of the course that were particularly helpful to me during pregnancy and subsequent labour was a session which concentrated on breathing. We were made to become aware of each other's breathing habits and our own. All of us were shallow and quick breathers but during the evening we all learned to improve our performance by breathing more slowly and deeply, and by exhaling more efficiently. During labour I was able to stay in control during long and painful contractions by concentrating on this method of breathing. During pregnancy breathing in this way must have been beneficial to the baby.

Becoming aware of ourselves and our movements, our position in time and space, meant recognizing the ungainly and often painful habits which we had acquired over many years. Learning to open a door with the other hand or to get up from the floor in a different way from our normal habit was quite a salutary experience. Most of us were unable to rise from a sitting position without thrusting our heads in the air, thereby putting strain on to our necks and spines. We learned how to use less muscular effort to stand, sit and walk, and were surprised at how little effort it actually takes to do any of these things.

In the later sessions we each received a 'treatment' during which our muscles were relaxed and unwound. Most of us 'grew' by an inch or two and I felt as light as air after leaving the couch, despite my enormous bump. Throughout my pregnancy I was totally free of backache. We learned to adopt a natural and comfortable sitting position without needing a chair-back for support; to stand and walk with as little muscular effort and strain as possible; and generally to adopt an ease of movement that would avoid muscular tension.

On 17th May my daughter was born with very little effort. The labour was approximately one hour, the second stage lasting about ten minutes. I needed no pain relief because due to concentrating on long slow breathing patterns and by drawing into myself as I have described earlier I was able to stay in complete control throughout. She is a happy, healthy little soul and I am constantly learning from her freedom and ease of movement.

I have only described here a few of the aspects of the Alexander Technique that have made such a very great impression on me. I can only add that I intend to continue learning from the Technique, not only on a physical level but as a basic philosophy of life.

CASE HISTORY

Alan Capel
Age: Thirty-nine
Occupation: Lorry-Driver

I left England in 1972 to hitch-hike to Australia. I was unencumbered by either a map or enough money, but with sufficient direction to get me there. It took four months in all, and it wasn't for another two years that I returned home. I was soon to move away from London and settle in south Devon.

Once there, I started my own haulage business delivering hay, straw and turf around the lovely Devon countryside. I moved into a flat with two friends who were surfing enthusiasts – an infection I was soon to catch. I bought my first board early in 1975, and by the end of the summer I was well and truly hooked.

Ten years and many waves later, the truck I drove for my living had grown to over eighteen metres in length; instead of the hundred-and-fifty bales of straw that my first truck had carried, this £20,000 Swedish vehicle carried eight hundred! At the end of another long hard summer season the truck was still going strong . . . but I was not. By October 1985 I had completely seized up.

What had started as a 'nuisance' pain behind my right knee turned into chronic sciatica which caused a pain that stretched from the base of my lumbar spine right down to my toes. The result of this caused my toes to curl under my foot making it difficult and painful to walk and, more importantly, I was unable to drive the truck.

Being a surfer I was an optimist, and I wasn't insured for such an event. My whole life ethic of 'work hard, play hard' was suddenly thrown back in my face, and to my ever-growing bewilderment I did not know why. All the people I turned to for help did not know either.

No work . . . let alone surf. No football. No achievement. No pride. No satisfaction. No fulfilment. No justification for the pain – just the endless throbbing which was robbing me of my life energy.

My eldest son Daniel, then three years old, did not understand why his dad could not rough and tumble with him, and with the arrival of his younger brother in the January of 1986 I was desperately seeking the answer to my problem. Within six weeks of the birth of Matthew I was admitted into Exeter's Orthopaedic Hospital for the 'final solution' – the removal of a prolapsed intervertebral disc pressing on the sciatic nerve at the base of my spine.

Two weeks later I was back at home in a worse state than ever, having been told by my surgeon that my discs were fine. Whilst there was no doubt in the consultant's mind that I was in considerable pain, he could offer me no solution to its cause as his knowledge was exhausted.

Doctors, osteopaths, physiotherapists, acupuncturists, consultants, nurses, surgeons and even faith healers had all done their best but to no avail . . . I was running out of options.

It was at this point that a friend recommended a course of lessons in the Alexander Technique. She was very sincere but I could hardly face yet another alternative health scheme even by well-meaning people.

I started having lessons mainly because I could not think of what else to do. There were no overnight miracles, but I was not expecting any. After fifteen lessons real changes started to happen; changes that not only led to a reduction in pain, but changes on levels that I never knew existed. Make no mistake, the Alexander Technique belongs in the realms of re-education in how you use both your body and your mind. The Technique has given me the opportunity to lose some of the harmful habits that were at the root of my sciatica, and has enabled me to get back into the driving seat of my own life. Real free choice is back in my hands once again.

CASE HISTORY

Joyce Ellis
Age: Sixty-seven
Occupation: Teacher

I had always been very fit up until the age of fifty-eight when severe back pain arose out of the blue. The pain extended from my lower back right down my right leg and even into my foot and toes. X-rays revealed scoliosis (abnormal curvature of the spine) which had produced premature wear and tear of the fourth and fifth lumbar vertebrae. The pain was relieved only when I was wearing a back brace, which temporarily and artificially improved my posture.

After retiring at the age of sixty-two I had two years with little pain and I stopped wearing the brace. Then to my dismay the pain returned worse than ever, only this time it was down my left leg. Although both my husband and son were doctors they were powerless to help, apart from giving me pain-killing drugs that didn't really solve the problem. I was forced to use a walking-stick which I hated, and the back brace no longer gave me the relief it used to. I was injected with anti-inflammatory agents under a general anaesthetic. Any further treatment was the removal of the damaged discs and even this drastic step did not ensure success.

I was determined to avoid this operation at all costs. My life had been completely disrupted; I even had to sleep downstairs because of my restricted mobility. My confidence had reached an all-time low; I did not know where to turn next.

It was at this point that I became aware of the Alexander Technique. I began to attend a class at the local technical college and also had some individual sessions. Within weeks my mobility had improved beyond recognition, and I had regained confidence in myself. With reasonable care my life has returned to normal. The stress that was induced by my illness has disappeared and has been replaced with the long-forgotten optimism that I had once enjoyed. Much to my surprise, my eyesight has significantly improved, and my blood pressure has lowered due to the more relaxed approach to life that I have adopted. This radically different way of being has not only affected my physical condition, but has also enhanced my relationships with friends and family.

This improved mental attitude has almost been of more use than the improvement in my mobility and the relative freedom from pain especially in view of my increasing age. The need to adapt mentally to the fact that I am unable to do as much as I used to has been very beneficial. In my life I have found that the Alexander Technique has given me the freedom to choose wisely as well as having provided me with a sound philosophy for living.

CASE HISTORY

Caroline Green
Age: Twenty-seven
Occupation: Computer
programmer/analyst

When I discovered the Alexander Technique early this year, I had been suffering from intermittent lower back pain and neck ache for some years, even at my relatively young age. I could not understand what it was that was causing the problem. I ate well, meditated regularly and even practised T'ai chi (a Chinese body and movement awareness technique), so I was convinced that I had retained a reasonable posture. I had also become aware over recent years that my breathing was often shallow and fast, and that there was a basic lack of ease throughout my whole body. However, awareness alone did not eradicate the problem, so nothing changed and I began to feel stuck. What I had failed to consider was that my lifestyle and my attitude to life could be part of the problem.

I had been brought up in a family of six. I had always done well at school and was expected to achieve a glowing career when I grew up . . . after all wasn't money and success the only way to lasting happiness? I went from school to college and then on to university and ended up with a BA in philosophy and an MSc in computing. I had never been taught to explore my own interests to see where they might lead. I grew up, like so many other people, believing that success and money were the two most important things in life, even at the cost of just being myself. I was heading for promotion after promotion in my job as a computer analyst, but where was this happiness that I had been promised for so long? I was becoming more and more miserable as the days went by because I was trying to be someone else rather than just myself.

Having tried a variety of complementary health therapies, I heard about the Alexander Technique. I started to have some lessons and was amazed at the remarkable effect of the few gentle movements that my teacher went through with me. I went away from my first lesson feeling light, free of tension and more full of energy than I had for a long time. He told me that this was how my body could feel if it were not so bound up with the physical tension resulting from harmful postural habits. I quickly realized that these habits had been caused by the unhealthy emotional and psychological attitudes that had been imposed on me by society. I noticed that I had a very persistent habit of slumping when I sat and that my shoulders were curving in towards each other – this was caused by a basic lack of confidence that had been with me through my childhood. As I began to expand the upper part of my chest I automatically began to have more confidence in myself; and after subsequent lessons there were many other psychological changes that went hand in hand with the physical ones.

I have begun to understand how my body works, and when I feel pain I recognize it as a signal for me to stop and listen to what it is trying to tell me. I have learned how to perform even simple tasks in a different way so as not to put undue stress on myself. I still suffer from a little back pain from time to time, but I can now eradicate it in a matter of minutes by lying in the recommended position. It was a revelation to me that I did not have to be a victim of pain and I could do something for myself to get rid of it. I no longer accept tension and pain as inevitable, and this makes me feel much more in control of my life.

I have come to realize that society had encouraged me to wear a 'strait-jacket' of fixed posture – I can still hear my teachers telling me to sit up straight with my shoulders back and stomach in. I know that they had the best of intentions and simply did not realize the great harm they were doing. I have also re-evaluated my idea of success and changed those things in my life that stopped me being myself.

I now work as a freelance computer technician/tutor and consultant and I love the challenge of inventing ideas rather than following those of other people. Looking back now at my previous office job, I can see that I was always accepting unreasonable deadlines and demands because I lacked basic confidence. The pace of life in the computer world is fast and furious. It is hard to retain one's peace of mind within that environment unless you stop from time to time to assess the ever-changing situation. I'm sorry to say this rarely happens, with the result that many millions of pounds are wasted each year.

In short, the benefits that I have so far received from having Alexander lessons are a dramatic improvement in my backache and neck tension, an increased level of happiness in my life, a greater sense of freedom, an increase in my confidence, and an ability to make real choices in my life. These benefits not only apply to my working life, but also spill over into my relationships with my friends and family.

CASE HISTORY

Susan Pearce
Age: Seventeen
Occupation: Student

About two years ago I was on the verge of going into hospital for a major operation. It had recently been confirmed that I was suffering from both scoliosis (a deformed curvature of the spine where the spine is bent either to the left or right), and lordosis (an unnatural forward curvature of spine). In fact my spine was curved as much as forty-four degrees.

Amazingly enough I was in no physical pain, but psychologically it affected my whole life. Other children at school were very cruel and I was nick-named 'the hunchback'. I used to cry myself to sleep nearly every night thinking about my problem. The other girls at school were all starting to have boyfriends and I was beginning to feel very isolated and alone.

I was told by the specialist that if nothing had changed in three months they would take me into hospital for an operation. The operation consisted of placing a metal rod down my back to help straighten it; I would have to be in plaster for six months at least. I was terrified.

My mother heard about the Alexander Technique through a friend who had been having lessons herself. At first I was sceptical, but I was willing to give anything a try.

Because of the severity of my condition, I was initially asked to come three times a week. Very soon I noticed that my balance and co-ordination had improved due to the fact that I was releasing a lot of muscular tension in my legs and feet – tension that I had previously been unaware of. Slowly I began to understand what I could do for myself. It had been very confusing at first, but then suddenly it all made sense.

After three months I was due to go back for further X-rays and both my doctors were amazed at the results that they saw. My condition had improved remarkably, and my hump was very much smaller as I was walking in a much more upright way. The scoliosis was also very much improved and today is hardly noticeable. Needless to say my operation was cancelled, much to my relief, and I am leading a normal life which would have been extremely unlikely two years ago.

CASE HISTORY

Wendy Wright
Age: Forty
Occupation: Physical education teacher

From an early age I had always been keen on sport, any sport – netball, basketball, athletics. As a child I thrived on it, and when it came to choosing a career sport was foremost in my mind.

I thoroughly enjoyed my job as a physical education teacher, and I very much missed it when I was forced to give it up twelve years ago to have my first child. I missed the excitement, the thrill, the ecstasy of the game. Something happened to my body whenever I played basketball, tennis, or simply ran. I would feel alive, free, and on top of the world. I would often wonder why I could not experience this feeling while going about my everyday activities (which more often than not were boring and mundane). I was often depressed in my day-to-day life, but never when I was playing sports. I had heard of the Alexander Technique briefly in passing, but when a friend of mine was helped to become free of pain when doctors and drugs had failed I began to become very curious.

So it was curiosity that made me seek out my first teacher. I did not have any aches or pains so I thought that maybe it would be a waste of time, but there was just a chance that this could help me recreate that feeling that I had so often experienced on the court. 'Maybes' were not enough for me. I had to know.

My life was very busy at that point in my life; I had three young children so I could no longer spare the time needed to play in leagues. Training and matches were eating up my precious time . . . time I should be spending with my young children. The more time I spent with my children, however, the more desperately I missed the feelings of freedom and exhilaration that went with playing sport.

I threw all my expectations of the Technique to the wind and walked into my first lesson. And I came away feeling freer and lighter than I had done for a long time.

As the lessons progressed I would feel happy and relaxed at times, and confused and angry at others. After all, who was this person telling me that I was using my leg muscles to excess? After all, I had been running and teaching running for many years. I needed to use these muscles and in this way! I remember leaving one of the lessons fuming with anger, but as I walked over to my car my annoyance subsided and was replaced with that feeling I had only been able to experience while running.

From that day on I have not looked back. Even though that particular feeling only lasted a couple of hours on that occasion, it showed me what was possible.

Today the Alexander Technique has become an integral part of my life. It has helped me as a mother, wife, and teacher. To me the Technique is not something esoteric, nor is it some strange appendix or addition to ordinary experience. It is not just a luxury for the rich. It pertains to the very structure of human consciousness and to the process of understanding oneself fully – which is each and everyone's birthright.

FURTHER READING

Brennan, R. *The Alexander Technique Manual*, Little Brown, 1996.

Brennan, R. *Health Essentials: The Alexander Technique*, Element Books, 1991.

Stevens, C. *Alexander Technique*, Optima, 1987.
These are easy-to-read books for people who know little or nothing about the Technique.

Gelb, M. *Body Learning*, Aurum Press, 1981.
An excellent follow-up book to any of the introductory books.

Barlow, W. *The Alexander Principle*, Gollancz, 1973.
Wilfred Barlow is a specialist in the National Health Service as well as a teacher of the Technique. This is an interesting book with an emphasis on the medical aspects of the Technique.

Westfeldt, L. F. *Matthias Alexander: The Man and His Work*, Centerline Press, 1986.
This is the autobiography of a polio victim who was helped to overcome her difficulty in walking, and then trained as an Alexander teacher. A very readable and often moving book.

Macdonald, P. *The Alexander Technique As I See It*, Rahula Books, 1989.
A collection of some interesting notebook jottings, which would be of special interest to people already involved in the Technique. Patrick Macdonald was one of the most experienced teachers in recent years, and was trained by Alexander himself.

Alexander, F. M. *The Use of the Self*
Alexander, F. M. *Man's Supreme Inheritance*
Alexander, F. M. *Constructive Conscious Control*
Alexander, F. M. *The Universal Constant in Living*
These books are of great value although they are not easy to read. You will probably need a dictionary to decipher many of the sentences.

Useful Addresses

Richard Brennan runs a three year teacher training course in Galway, Ireland, as well as shorter weekend and week courses in Ireland and UK. For details of any of these courses please send a s.a.e. to:

The Alexander Technique Training Centre
c/o Richard Brennan
13 Bru Na Mara
Fort Lorenzo
Galway
Eire

For a list of teachers in your area please contact one of the following addresses:

UNITED KINGDOM

The Society of Teachers of the Alexander Technique
20 London House, 266 Fulham Road
London SW10 9EL

Alexander Technique International
142 Thorpedale Road
London N4 3BS

DENMARK

The South African Society of Teachers of the Alexander Technique
Wergelandsalle 21
DK-2660
Soborg

FRANCE

Alexander Technique International
c/o Steketee
25 rue Pradier
75019 Paris

THE NETHERLANDS

The Netherlands Society of Teachers of the Alexander Technique
Max Haverlaarlaan 80
1183 HN Amstelveen

SWEDEN

Stralgatan 2 (11)
11263 Stockholm

SWITZERLAND

The Swiss Society of Teachers of the Alexander Technique
Postfach
CH 8032
Zurich

USA

Alexander Technique International, Inc.
1692 Massachusetts Avenue
3rd Floor
Cambridge, MA 02138

The North American Society of Teachers of
the Alexander Technique
PO Box 112484
Tacoma
WA 98411-2484

Alexander Technique Workshops (USA)
PO Box 408
Ojai
California 93024

CANADA

The Canadian Society of Teachers of the
Alexander Technique
Box 47025
Apt. 12
555 West 12th Avenue
Vancouver
BC V5Z 3X0

SOUTH AFRICA

The South African Society of Teachers of the
Alexander Technique
35 Thornhill Road
Rondesbosch 7700

AUSTRALIA

The Australia Society of Teachers of the
Alexander Technique
PO Box 716
Darlinghurst
NSW 2010

Alexander Technique International
11/11 Stanley Street
Darlinghurst
NSW 2010

Direction Magazine
(A Journal on the Alexander Technique with
world-wide subscriptions)
PO BOX 276
Bondi
NSW 2026

THE ALEXANDER SELF HELP TAPE

This is the perfect accompaniment to the Alexander Technique Manual and gives clear and
concise instructions on:

- How to eliminate unwanted tension.
- How to prevent or relieve back pain.
- How to improve your breathing.
- How to clear your mind from unwanted thoughts.
- How to practice the two Alexander principles of Inhibition and Direction.
- How to stay in the present moment.

This audio cassette is available from:

Richard Brennan, 13 Bru Na Mara, Fort Lorenzo, Galway, Eire and is priced **£9.99**

RESIDENTIAL COURSES ON THE ALEXANDER TECHNIQUE

DORSET

Gaunts House
Wimborne
Dorset BH21 4JQ
Tel: 0202 841522

Monkton Wyld Court
Charmouth
Bridport
Dorset DT6 6DQ
Tel: 0297 60342

SPAIN

Cortijo Romero
c/o 24 Grange Avenue
Chapletown
Leeds
Yorkshire LS7 4EJ
Tel: 0532 374015

GREECE

(Two week residential course)
The Skyros Institute
Skyros
92 Prince of Wales Road
London NW5 2NE

NON-RESIDENTIAL COURSES AND INDIVIDUAL SESSIONS IN LONDON

The Highbury Centre
137 Grovesnor Avenue
Highbury
London N5 2NH
Tel: 071 226 5805

THE ALEXANDER TECHNIQUE SELF-HELP TAPE

This is the perfect accompaniment to *The Alexander Technique Workbook* and gives clear and concise instructions on:

● How to relieve unwanted tension
● How to prevent or relieve back pain
● How to improve your breathing
● How to clear your mind from unwanted thoughts
● How to practice the two Alexander principles of Direction and Inhibition.
● How to stay in the present moment

This audio cassette is available from The Alexander Centre, 12 Brooklands, Totnes, Devon TQ9 5AR, and is priced **£7.99** (inc p&p).

INDEX